Human Security in China

Chi Zhang
Editor

Human Security in China

A Post-Pandemic State

palgrave
macmillan

Editor
Chi Zhang
St Andrews, UK

ISBN 978-981-16-4674-4 ISBN 978-981-16-4675-1 (eBook)
https://doi.org/10.1007/978-981-16-4675-1

This Palgrave Macmillan imprint is published by the registered company Springer Nature Singapore Pte Ltd.
The registered company address is: 152 Beach Road, #21-01/04 Gateway East, Singapore 189721, Singapore

Acknowledgements

The idea of applying the concept of human security comes from my Ph.D. supervisor Edward Newman. His expertise, experience and encouragement inspired and continue to inspire me to pursue knowledge and challenge conventional wisdom. Conceived during the pandemic, this volume did not arise from an in-person conference, where synergies take place naturally. The contributors of all chapters showed particular dedication and professionality to put together this interdisciplinary effort.

The ideas for this book have been presented at the Political Studies Association Annual Conference on 31 March and Royal Irish Academy Annual conference on 29 April 2021. We thank the organisers, panel chairs and participants for offering pertinent feedback on this volume.

We are grateful to the Palgrave Macmillan editorial team, especially Balaji Varadharaju and Aurelia Heumader for their help throughout the publishing process. We are in debt of Jacob Dreyer for seeing value in the project and shepherding it through to completion. We thank anonymous reviewers who offered encouraging and helpful comments on this project.

Special thanks go to the British Academy (2020–2023) for funding my postdoctoral fellowship, which allows me to spend time on coordinating this project. This book also benefited immensely from the School of International Relations and the Handa Centre for the Study of Terrorism and Political Violence at the University of St Andrews, and the lovely colleagues who are always extremely supportive.

Many people have contributed, knowingly or unknowingly, to the development of this volume. We are grateful to them for their time, generosity, and intellect. All errors and shortcomings are my own.

Contents

Notes on Contributors

Dr Geoffrey C. Chen is an Associate Professor at the Department of China Studies, School of Humanities and Social Sciences at Xi'an Jiaotong-Liverpool University in Suzhou, China. His current research focuses on energy security, environmental politics, and the international political economy of energy. He is the author of *Governing Sustainable Energies in China* (Palgrave Macmillan, 2016) and co-author with David Toke, Antony Froggatt and Richard Connolly of *Nuclear Power in Stagnation: A Cultural Approach to Failed Expansion* (Routledge, 2021).

Dr. Hai Guo is an assistant research fellow at the Institute of Public Policy (IPP), South China University of Technology. His research focuses on East Asian politics and psychological theory in international relations. Prior to joining IPP, Guo received his Ph.D. from the University of Leeds, where he wrote a thesis on the "history problem" in Sino-Japanese relations between 1982 and 2012. He is currently working on various research projects, including a book on the history of Chinese diplomacy.

Jinru Huang is a Ph.D. candidate studying educational development and the accountability mechanism in China's education system at the Centre for Global Development (CDG), School of Politics and International Studies, University of Leeds. Huang did his field research in Ningxia (Muslim) Hui Autonomous Region, China in 2020, and his research also has a focus on the education of China's ethnic minorities.

Dr. Catherine Jones is a lecturer at the University of St Andrews, Scotland (UK). Previously she was the East Asia Research Fellow at the University of Warwick from 2012–2018. She received her Ph.D. from the University of Reading. Her current research explores the nexus between security and development in East Asia. She has numerous publications including a monograph on 'China's challenge to liberal norms' (Palgrave 2019), an edited volume China and North Korea between Development and Security (Edward Elgar), as well as a range of journal articles and book chapters including Defining Taiwan Out (Contemporary Politics), Contesting within Order? China, socialisation and practice (Cambridge Review of International Affairs).

Dr. Jia Liu is an assistant research fellow at the Institute of Public Policy (IPP), South China University of Technology. Her main research interests are global justice related to extreme poverty as well as public health law. She has experience in jurisprudential research and social-legal studies. Her current research project focuses on socio-legal aspects of China's public health management system. Her work on global justice appears in *Asian Legal Philosophy, Chinese (Taiwan) Review of International and Transnational Law*, etc.

Dr. Qiyang Liu is a research fellow at Peking University. He received Ph.D. from the Institute for Transport Studies, University of Leeds in 2019. His research interests include transport policy in the Global South, policy transfer, and transport-related social inequities. His work has been published in leading journals in the transport field, such as *Transport Policy*.

Dr. Chi Zhang is a British Academy Postdoctoral Fellow at the University of St Andrews and an Associate Member of the Handa Centre for the Study of Terrorism and Political Violence. Her areas of research interest fall broadly within security studies, constructivism and Chinese political philosophy. She holds a Ph.D. in Politics and International Studies from the University of Leeds, and a master's degree in South Asian Area Studies from the School of Oriental and African Studies. She published in *Terrorism and Political Violence, Studies in Conflict & Terrorism, Politics and Religion* and*Asian Security*.

Dr. Qian Zhang is a health psychologist who has gained a doctorate degree from the University of Leeds, UK. Her research interests focus on understanding determinants of health behaviour and investigating effective strategies for behaviour change. She is particularly interested in promoting health behaviour change using advanced digital technologies such as mobile apps and social media. She is also interested in promoting mental health and behaviour change using mindfulness-based approaches.

List of Figures

List of Tables

CHAPTER 1

Introduction

Chi Zhang

2020 was a year of disasters. It is through disasters that our lack of human-centred security is made apparent. In seeking to make sense of a post-pandemic world the concept of human security has gained particular traction and academic leverage. COVID-19 offers a unique chance to probe into the changing concept of security. Among chronic threats inherited from the past, such as hunger, disease and repression, and apocalyptic environmental degradation, be it abnormally heavy rain in Africa, biblical locust swarms and unprecedented fire in Australia, COVID-19 is perhaps unique, not only because this particular type of coronavirus is something that humanity has never seen, but because it has brought such a profound shock to the world of globalisation as we know it, and accelerates the process of de-globalisation that has already taken a foothold since the 2008 financial crisis and in the context of the US's withdrawal from its global leadership role during the Trump administration. In this regard, COVID-19 differentiates itself from any previous public health crises, such as the 1918 Spanish flu, SARS, MERS and Ebola. Yet from another perspective, COVID-19 may not be so unique. The pandemic

C. Zhang (✉)
St Andrews, UK
e-mail: cz38@st-andrews.ac.uk

C. Zhang (ed.), *Human Security in China*,
https://doi.org/10.1007/978-981-16-4675-1_1

has exposed and exacerbated the existing vulnerabilities that have threatened the experience of security at the individual level since antiquity. A glance at the human security literature reveals the friction between state security and human security, even in peaceful times and peaceful regions. As the 1994 Human Development Report, the pioneering articulation of the concept, insightfully points out, '[f]or most people today, a feeling of insecurity arises more from worries about daily life than from the dread of a cataclysmic world event' (UNDP 1994, 3). This observation made almost three decades ago still holds true today.

As global attention is focussed on the pandemic of the COVID-19 and its impacts on various aspects of life, considerable efforts are being made to summarise the lessons learned from different countries, among which China stands out as the country in which the first known cases was reported, the most extreme lockdowns were carried out and social order has been brought back under control, albeit not without costs, by a powerful central government. This global crisis invited us to reflect on the relationship between state security and human security in a time of unprecedented international connectedness. The concept of human security is a helpful analytical tool to probe into the question that is at the core of this pandemic: to what extent does the change of the reference object from the 'state' to 'human' affect the balance between individual freedom and the well-being of the wider community in practice?

The Predicament of Human Security: Criticality vs Practicality

Initially emerging as a policy concept in the 1994 UNDP Human Development Report, Human Security comes with an inherent dilemma (Newman 2017, 28). As a concept that emphasises individuals and communities as the referent object and beneficiary of security (Newman 2010, 78), Human Security[1] has been used in various international policy settings. Through the Human Security Network funded by Canada and Norway in 1998, human security has been embedded into the international norms and security agenda (Chinkin and Kaldor 2017, 504). While the use of the concept within the UN is often criticised as ambiguous and

[1] In this edited volume, the capitalised 'Human Security' is used to refer to the doctrine of Human Security applied by, for example, UN and EU, while 'human security' is referred to generally as a concept.

lacking substance, the UN's role in facilitating an ideational change from state-centric security to population-centred security cannot be ignored (MacFarlane and Khong 2006, 9).

At the regional level, in 2003, the concept of human security was proposed as a distinctive policy identity and posture to command consensus within the EU (Martin and Kaldor 2009, 160). At the fortieth anniversary of the Association of Southeast Asian Nations (ASEAN), the phrase 'people-oriented ASEAN' in the ASEAN Charter marked a 'human security' turn within Southeast Asia (Nishikawa 2010, 30). Explicitly or implicitly, East Asian countries, including Thailand, the Philippines, Japan and China began to incorporate the idea of human security into their security policies (Hernandez et al. 2019, 8). Regional organisations in Africa have worked towards crystalising human rights commitments into practices. For example, the Treatment Action Campaign of South Africa contributed to including HIV/AIDS in the human security agenda (Sabi and Rieker 2017).

Despite the universal recognition of the importance of human security, its potential to erode state sovereignty prevented it from being widely adopted. While countries like Canada, Japan and Norway were initially quick to embrace the concept,[2] the US, Russia and China 'resist the replacement or supplementation of state security by human security' (MacFarlane and Khong 2006, 10).

Like many radical ideas, human security started as an idea to challenge the traditional paradigm of security studies that centred around the survival of the state. This idea prompted scholars and practitioners to reconceptualise the provider and receiver of security as public goods. At the same time, like many radical ideas, human security has been used loosely and superficially by traditionalist foreign policy bureaucrats (Krause 2014). The conception has been overstretched and diluted by its own broadened scope and the accompanying vagueness, the consequence of which would be the 'securitisation' of any issues that were newly included in the security agenda (Christie 2014, 103). The very process of securitisation reinforced the power of the state as it is often the state which decides what constitutes a security threat (Christie 2014, 103).

[2] Even these countries became hesitant to adopt the concept, evident from Canada's withdrawal from advocacy and use of the concept, see Mary and Taylor's 'The second generation of human security: lessons from the UN and EU experience'.

Reflected in policy circles, the friction between 'criticality' and 'practicality' is manifested in various policy scenarios. A study of the security policy of the EU demonstrates how the vagueness of the concept prevents it from passing the 'reality check' (Matlary 2008, 132). The overuse of the rhetoric of human security makes its implementation ethically questionable, as calling all the EU security policy 'human security' only 'promises more than policy can deliver' (Matlary 2008, 143). The disappointment reached a point where human security is considered beyond redemption, as 'it has been institutionalized and co-opted to work in the interests of global capitalism, militarism and neoliberal governance' (Albrecht et al. 2007, 3).

In this sense, human security has been 'recuperated', borrowing the term from situationists, in which process critical ideas associated with Human Security are no longer challenging, but have been neutralised and absorbed into 'the existing political, legal and normative constraints of the "real world"' (Newman 2017, 28). The 'uncomfortable duality' of being both intellectually challenging and policy-relevant (Newman 2014, 227) makes it difficult to move human security forward and to rejuvenate itself beyond a 'vague amorphous add-on to harder-edged areas of security such as military or states security' (James 2014, 73). Paradoxically, radical ideas challenging the orthodox provide opportunities for the present officialdom to fine-tune their mechanism of control (Gardiner 2009, 227). Giving interventions a 'feel-good' name of human security may improve the coherence of a security paradigm, but 'interventions rarely happen for human security reasons alone' (Matlary 2008, 143). The wars in Afghanistan and Iraq, fought in the name of promoting human rights and democracy, illustrate how the notion of 'human rights' can be 'twisted and utilized to bolster repressive forces' (Gardiner 2009, 233). The interventionist nature of human security concerns remains unchanged, and the frequent invocation of human security to justify intervention contributes to the de-legitimisation of the concept in 'a two-tiered global legal order, with a self-selected group of liberal states imposing, through force, their unilateral moral judgements onto weaker states outside of the consent-based UN legal framework' (Franceschet 2016, 35). Adopting the language of human security, the Northern governments effectively framed their interests in the Global South to justify broader liberal interventionist practices (Christie 2014, 99). The Western imposition of liberal values in the name of human security, in the light of the *realpolitik* unilateralism, is criticised as an extension of 'human rights imperialism' (Martin and Owen 2014, 11), evidenced by the UN-sanctioned intervention in Libya.

As the first-generation Liberal Peace model failed, evidenced by military interventions in the name of the War on Terror and Geo-Politics, Chinkin and Kaldor (2017, 479–80) highlight the relevance of second-generation human security as a 'rights-based approach to peace-making and intervention that is both top-down and bottom-up, both international and local, and that requires extensive political, economic, legal and security tools'. The notable retreat of Canada, a former advocate of the human security agenda, led to some serious reflections on the vagueness of the concept and its problematic institutionalisation as a policy paradigm (Martin and Owen 2010). The lessons regarding the implementation of Human Security, largely drawn from western experience, necessitate a need to broaden the context in which the concept of human security is applied to 'de-westernise' (on de-Westernisation, see Glück 2015) the research of security.

The above discussion over the predicament of human security demonstrates the difficulty in bringing the debate to a quick end. Indeed, the aim of this edited volume is not to locate an ultimate solution to any of the thorny questions regarding the balance between state security and human security, even though it is tempting to make a hasty conclusion out of the frustration with governments' inability to regulate the population in the middle of a global crisis.

While the discussion has been ongoing since 1994 (UNDP 1994), the pandemic in 2020 has made it unprecedently clear that peace without development is bound to be fragile, as less developed countries were hit most severely by the economic chaos, entrenched social divisions and intensified conflicts that accompanied the spread of the virus. The ongoing pandemic offers an interesting scenario to reconsider the impact of the idea of human security on governance. Albeit all the demerits of the concept of human security, there is no doubt that the conceptual leap has made its impact in facilitating serious considerations of individual well-being (MacFarlane and Khong 2006, 163). The rhetorical adoption does have consequences, as 'once states (and more importantly, bureaucrats within foreign policy apparatuses) come to regard "human security" as an appropriate label for what they are already doing, the discourse has triumphed' (Krause 2014, 83).

At a more profound level, the alleged clash between human security and state security reflects the intellectual concern about the relationship between sovereign power and biopolitics. The latter is different from the former as it concerns the population more than territory. 'It is about the "power to make live" rather than the "right to kill"' (Chinkin and Kaldor 2017, 516). The COVID-19 pandemic has accentuated the biopolitical nature of governance in contemporary politics. It has helped the states to define the conditions of exceptionality that allow sovereign power to authorise restrictions that would otherwise not be observed by the people. The case of the pandemic illustrates that the line between sovereign power and biopolitics can no longer be identified easily. It has forced the government to choose between public health and economic grown, between those who will die of COVID-19 and those who will die of lack of access to food or medical care during lockdowns, and between letting some patients die in quarantine camps and letting the whole population get infected. It has confronted the government with a trolly problem to which no solution can be justified impeccably. It has also highlighted the question of biopolitics that treats life as 'bare life', whereby the state disregards aspects of personhood and develops 'protocols of communication and administration that treat people as objects' (Edkins 2008, 212). In this context, the disorder has merely been managed or contained, rather than resolved, by development cloaked in benevolence with 'constant invocation of rights, freedom and the people' (Duffield 2007, i).

Human Security in China

Despite the plethora of research on human security, Chinese perspectives remain marginal. While there have been some efforts in making links between Chinese human security approach and the wider intellectual engagements that are taking place outside China, these efforts fall short in terms of critical engagement with the central normative paradox of human security as sketched out earlier (Tow et al. 2013; Cui 2019; Ren 2019).

The applicability of such an ideal as a 'post-liberal peace', using the language of Chinkin and Kaldor, in China is far from straightforward. To be sure, the idea of human security is not entirely alien to China (see Ren 2019). China has begun to develop a 'new concept of security' since the 1990s in response to the collapse of the Soviet Union and the end of the Cold War, the new reality in which military alliances and build-up of armaments do not lead to lasting peace (Thayer 2003, 89). Hu Jintao's elaboration on the concept highlights the broader international consensus on the need to reflect on the traditional security paradigm and indicates a different path China seeks to embark on that contrasts the interventionist undertone in the Human Security discourse.

> *A new security concept that embraces the principles of equality, dialogue, trust and cooperation, and a new security order should be established to ensure genuine mutual trust, mutual cooperation, consensus through consultation, and peaceful settlement of disputes, rather than bullying, confrontation, and imposition of one's own will upon others. Only in that way can countries coexist in amity and secure their development.* (quoted in Thayer 2000)

China continued to promote the New Security Concept in the aftermath of the 9/11 attacks, using the practice of the Shanghai Cooperation Organisation as a 'successful case' (Ministry of Foreign Affairs 2002). Targeting Southeast Asian neighbours, the New Security Concept did not fully achieve its intended goal of counteracting the US presence in the region. However, the development of New Security Concept signals a departure from the unilateral, sovereign-centric security outlook under early leaders of the Chinese Communist Party (CCP) and to a multilateral, people-oriented approach under Hu. 'People-oriented governance' or 'people-centred approach' became an important part of Hu's vision of a 'harmonious society' that 'puts people first' (*yirenweiben*) (Ren 2019, 56). While China's interpretation of R2P is relatively conservative (see Zheng 2016), focussing on capacity-building (Pillar I) more than intervention (Pillar 3), Beijing's participation in the discussion and application of R2P ensured its role in international norm-shaping (Foot 2011). Nevertheless, the problem with this concept did not go unnoticed, even in China. Chinese scholars join critics of Human Security in questioning the excessively broadened scope that rendered the concept meaningless (Han 2000; He 2004), and acknowledge the predicament of human security in China in terms of income, health, pension, environment and poverty (by Hu Angang, cited in Chapter 4).

A more recent version of China's security concept, the 'Overall Security Outlook', is promoted by Xi Jinping as a set of all-encompassing tenets that govern all aspects of security governance. Xi stresses the importance of a 'people-oriented' and 'human-oriented' security approach, requiring the officials to 'adhere to the principle that national security serves the people, relies on the people, and truly achieve a solid foundation for national security' (Xi 2014). The emphasis on the masses is consistent with Xi's efforts to revive the Mass Line ethos that shored up legitimacy in the Mao era. In support of the Overall Security Outlook, Chinese scholars developed theories that seek to differ China's security model from, and complement, if not challenge, Western ones. These theories include 'sustainable security' by Liu Jiangyong (2017) and 'harmonism' (*hehe zhuyi*) by Yu Xiaofeng, who borrows the concept from the *Book of Changes* (2018). Other attempts to reconceptualise 'security' are part of the broader efforts of the Chinese IR scholars to introduce Chinese political philosophy into the understanding of China's changing position in the international system, which include 'creative involvement' by Wang Yizhou (2017), 'moral realism' by Yan Xuetong (see, for example, Paltiel 2011), 'relationality and processual construction' by Qin Yaqing (2009), the 'new tianxia system' by Zhao Tingyang (2006). While the promise of a 'people-oriented' approach is considered largely rhetorical and 'problem-solving', using the language of Robert Cox, the burgeoning literature on human security in China illustrates that the CCP can no longer afford to disregard individuals and communities when it is seeking to achieve the stated goal of 'collective security' (Xi 2013).

China's developmental approach to security, in theory, echoes the 'development as freedom' thesis by Amartya Sen. Zhong Feiteng, a researcher at the Chinese Academy of Social Sciences, conceptualises China's approach to security that came into shape in the Deng era as 'developmental security' (Zhong 2015, 116). According to Zhong, this approach not only emphasises the parallel importance of development and military/political security, but also determines the priority of different security concerns and how resources should be distributed. 'Developmental security' also highlights that development is the precondition of state security, and military modernisation, as a means to security, should serve the ends of economic development strategy and security strategy. Although this approach refrains from using 'rights' and 'freedom', words that bear direct connotations to individualistic values originated in the West, it shares the goal of the Human Security agenda of improving the well-being of the people.

Despite the rhetorical commitment, the idea of human security acquired some problems in practice, just like other imported ideas that have been sinicised (*zhongguohua*) into the political language in China (Breslin 2015).

When applying the concept of human security to China, and more widely East Asian context, a new level of analysis emerges. Chinese culture draws heavily on the Confucian tradition that emphasises collective interests (see Breslin 2015). Although throughout history, when Confucianism was endorsed by the state, collective interests were often co-opted, and collectivism has been deeply embedded in East Asian societies to mediate between the individual and the state. Thus, the individual/state dualism that dominates the human security debate must be adapted to include collectivism for a meso-level analysis. The community level human security is analysed in Chapters 3, 5 and 6.

The CCP's vision of security is conceived within the framework of collective interests that can only be guaranteed with a capable central government, the absence of which invites regional powers fighting for control, leading to a far worse situation in which individual human security would be unthinkable. The empowerment of individuals is only possible under the prerequisite of a powerful central government that ensures the stability of its territories. The fear of 'chaos' (*luan*) and the obsession with 'stability' (*wending*) have dictated the CCP's approaches to civil disobedience and separatist movements, most vividly captured by Deng's slogan 'stability overrides everything'. This mentality continues to dictate the CCP's approach to the pandemic, manifested by the Letter of Reprimand by the Wuhan police that admonishes the whistle-blower doctor Li Wenliang for his warning against the coronavirus in December 2019. This mentality perpetuates the existing power relations by maintaining dissent at a minimum level. The rhetorical commitment to human security backfires when people do not feel their interests are sufficiently represented. One does not need to dig deep to see how state-sponsored ideas like 'harmonious society' were ridiculed in China. Dissent may have been 'harmonised' (*bei hexie*), or censored, online, but it continued to exist in forms of irony and satire that mock state propaganda and censorship (see Nordin and Richaud 2014; Wang et al. 2016; Callahan 2012). Not only was China's 'human security' questioned domestically, but its international aid was also criticised for serving its economic interests (Cui 2019, 156).

Research Question

The discussions about the criticality/practicality conundrum and the *sinicised* human security in China beg the question: **to what extent does 'human security' as a concept, norm and a set of discourses facilitate China's shift from a nation-based security governance approach to an individual-based approach, albeit within the constraint of a 'national human security' model?** Within the institutional constraints in China, the human security agenda has to 'dance in shackles', making its way towards recuperation or obliviation at the whim of the central authority. The defenders of human security have to work within the constraints of the given reality in which the structural sources of deprivation can hardly be changed (see Newman 2016a, 1167).

China is but one example of the countries in the world whose 'practice of human security is still largely state-centric, piecemeal and protection-oriented' (Hernandez et al. 2019, 9). However, in the context of COVID-19, China is selected as a testing ground for theoretical engagement with the concept of human security for three reasons. First, the relatively high level of mass support albeit its regime type warrants special attention in the context of COVID-19, as this pandemic is particularly good at eroding legitimacy by exposing existing weaknesses of the government. China serves as a valuable case study to understand the relationship between the governments' commitment to human security and regime type. What the CCP calls 'institutional superiority' and institutional constraints of an authoritarian state can enhance our knowledge about similarities and differences in the states' approaches to the pandemic.

Second, the ongoing pandemic has put the relative decline of the US and the relative rise of China under the spotlight. With the US recovering from Trumpism and China advancing in global governance, it is important to examine the impact this shifting relationship is having on the international norms of human security. A good way to start is by looking at the ideas and practices of human security within China, in combination with its rhetorical commitment to human security on multilateral platforms such as the UN and ASEAN.

Third, although Chinese intellectuals have not been engaging in the concept of human security and critical security studies in the same way as their Western counterparts have, to ensure regime survival, the

Chinese government has developed sophisticated mechanisms to co-opt the idea of human security into the agenda of national security, without adopting the exact language. While Chinese engagement with the concept of human security is not 'critical' in an academic sense, the pragmatistic co-optation of human security language is likely to put some constraints on its norms of security studies and policies. In interrogating this process, we challenge the existing security paradigm by unravelling the structural conditions that give rise to insecurity. The China case also contributes to the debate about the Copenhagen School's critique of human security. Although the state power is further strengthened by lengthening the list of security concerns, previous cases of epidemics—SARS and avian influenza—demonstrates that desecuritisation could be detrimental (Wishnick 2010). This approach thus offers insights in addressing the reconciliation between 'critical aspirations' and 'political realities' (Newman 2016a) from a less explored non-Western perspective.

This volume aims at going beyond listing relevant ideas and practices in China's security policies. It is an attempt to inform the broader debates about the analytical value of the concept and how to retain its criticality in a state in which reform can only be made by cooperating with the state. Edward Newman points out in a volume that juxtaposes the Chinese, Japanese and Australian approaches to human security, that 'the state remains the key reference for security in Asia and that any shift in the direction of human security will be towards 'national human security' (Newman 2016b, 214).

To make sense of the impact of the idea of human security in countries like China, human security cannot be thought of in black and white terms. Promoting human security in a state-monitored environment might risk neutralisation and absorption of resistance. However, it is only in coordination with a capable state can the idea of human security be brought to the attention of a wider audience. In other words, the challenge to the state must be constrained to the extent that radical ideas are allowed to enter public debate. While this balance is certainly tilted in favour of the state in China, we value the very existence of radical ideas and their critical, yet albeit limited, potential to make long-term changes to China's logic of governance. As Henri Lefebvre (2005) suggests, 'because a radical idea is vulnerable to recuperation does not mean it is itself recuperative' (cited in Gardiner 2009, 233). While the human security programmes in China remain largely rhetorical, state-sponsored and top-down, the incorporation of the idea of human security into everyday practices gives the people the ideational framework to understand their security at an individual or communal level. At the very least, the nationalist propaganda that celebrates an imposed victimhood caused by the alleged injustice of the US-led world order struggles to maintain its traction among those who were disillusioned by the government's failure to control the early spread of COVID-19 and its habitual attempts to silence dissent that might pose a challenge to 'stability maintenance' (*weiwen*).

Therefore, we draw on Edward Newman's definition of Human Security: '[i]n its broadest sense, "human security" seeks to place the individual—or people collectively—as the *referent* [emphasis in original] of security, rather than, although *not necessarily in opposition to* [emphasis added], institutions such as a territory and state sovereignty' (Newman 2001, 239). We are conscious of the limited ability of critical ideas to circumvent the powerful, as De Larrinaga and Doucet (2008, 517) observe through the case of War on Terror, 'the human security discourse informs the current biopolitical networks of world order and often works in conjunction with—rather than against—the global exercise of sovereign power…'.

Building on these theoretical insights, this volume examines how a state-led, top-down shift of the *referent* from the state to human—the *given reality of security* in China—reinvents the existing rules of the game, entrenches the established power relations, and neutralises radical critique of its state-centred approach. This is particularly reflected in Chapters 3, 5 and 6. At the same time, we also highlight that Human Security is not entirely hopeless, and in some cases, it does fuel bottom-up empowerment. Chapters 4 and 8 illustrate how radical ideas have been brought into public consciousness at the risk of recuperation.

The interdisciplinarity of this volume offers various perspectives that allow us to probe into different aspects of human security as it is being incorporated into China's security rhetoric. As COVID-19 as taken a foothold across the world, its impact has gone far beyond virology. Where it has spread, it has paralysed health systems, exacerbated existing tensions and divisions, eroded government legitimacy, induced endless blame games, and provoked xenophobia. Measures to contain it have caused economic recession, unemployment, the ensuing mass protests in relatively well-off countries, and interruption of humanitarian assistance to conflict-stricken regions. As it distracted attention from existing peace processes, states and non-state actors took this crisis as an opportunity to advance their political interests, evident from the Russia-Saudi oil war and the increasing level of conflict in Africa and the Middle East despite the UN call for a ceasefire. The multi-faceted nature of COVID-19 cannot be sufficiently explained without an interdisciplinary approach.

The marriage of human security and interdisciplinarity addresses the agenda of human security by entertaining interdisciplinary efforts to explore global vulnerabilities from previously under-researched perspectives in security studies. In doing so, this volume gives the discussion of the pandemic an overarching structure and analytical depth by contextualising it in the broader debate over human security. It is hoped that this will generate a sustained theoretical relevance in the aftermath of the COVID-19 crisis which is likely to have lasting effects on how people live.

Chapter Outline

The remainder of this edited volume is organised in eight subsequent chapters. Chapter 2 starts with China's changing role as represented in news media since the pandemic. The analysis of the narratives in international media about China reveals the gap between China's own rhetoric of 'human security' and 'responsibility' and the reception of such rhetoric in the international community. From an International Relations (IR) perspective, this chapter situates China's approach to people-centred security within the international efforts to define 'human' in the concept of human security. The gap highlights a shared theme that runs throughout this edited volume: that China's definition of 'human' leans more towards the community, the collective, the entire population, rather than the individual. Such a definition leads to positive and negative consequences in implementation, which are elaborated in the following chapters. Considering that there are certain 'Chinese characteristics' in China's approach to security, Jones teases out the differences between the use of term 'security', 'stability' and 'safety' in the implementation of these concepts.

As Jones rightly points out, China follows an approach of 'learning from doing' that allows it to be rhetorically pragmatic. This approach, in the context of human security, allows China to justify its distinctive pattern of behaviour in the UN Security Council that prioritises the agency of the state as the central actor in protecting.

This chapter usefully highlights that China's approach is not unique or isolated from the rest of the international community. Its rationale that gives more weight to collective human security over the individual level, as well as its emphasis on the agency of the state, are shared by others in the international community. Jones' conceptual map (Fig. 2.1) helpfully illustrates the relationship between different states' approaches. Drawing on the Responsibility to Protect (R2P) literature, Jones offers a powerful analytical framework (Table 2.1) that brings human security and R2P into conversation with each other.

Jones applies this analytical framework in examining how China's responses to the pandemic has been framed and represented in news media. One of the sources of divergence between China and the international community is the transparency of information. This aspect of China's approach has reinforced the unfavourable views that the international community holds about it. Despite the effectiveness of China's responses in controlling infections domestically, its commitment to human safety is not duly recognised in the news media examined in this chapter.

Overall, this chapter, drawing on the IR literature and comparative insights, lays a solid foundation for the following chapters to probe further into China's approach to human security in the following chapters.

Chapter 3 focuses on the legitimacy crisis following the early mishandling of the virus when it was reported in Wuhan. Drawing on the CCP's history of mass movements to improve the hygiene level, Guo contextualises public health as a key aspect of the CCP's commitment to human security, hence its key source of legitimacy. Through the 'party-state-society' triangle, Guo demonstrates how the CCP is inherently vulnerable to, and the mechanisms it has developed to cope with, legitimacy crises.

The 'party-state-society' captures the interactions between the state/central authority, local authorities and society. In a system where performance matters more than democratic procedure, accountability functions differently than in liberal democracies. The party-state-society triangle makes it possible for the state to manipulate the public's distrust with local authorities and use people's dissatisfaction in its favour.

Guo examines the 'upward accountability system' in which officials answer primarily to their superiors, rather than their constituencies. This institutional feature encourages officials to prioritise top-down orders over bottom-up information flow. Such a system disincentivises officials to share information about a potential crisis as doing so reflects badly on their performances, thus ruining their prospect for promotion. The early mishandling of the pandemic reveals how such a system resists change—while a web-based reporting system was developed following SARS in 2004, it was almost completely absent in reporting the COVID-19.

When local authorities failed to deliver good governance, the central authority stepped in, touting the 'fantasy for a benign patriarch' that aligned its interest with citizens, delivering justice for them and honouring the CCP's promises of providing society with security and stability. The way in which the CCP handled the legitimacy crisis following the COVID-19 pandemic has important implications for understanding how authoritarian regimes sustain its rule. Like liberal democracies, the CCP does commit to human security—although it did not use the same language, its history of mass mobilisations demonstrates its commitment regarding the well-being of the people. This chapter highlights how the CCP's commitment to human security, hence its legitimacy, has been undermined significantly during the pandemic, when many governments across the world have also been experiencing legitimacy crises. The 'party-state-society' demonstrates how the CCP is still able to defend its commitment to human security, by distancing itself from and deflecting blame to local authorities.

Chapter 4 offers a comprehensive analysis of the evolution of China's approach to alternative energy during COVID-19 with case studies of three emerging sectors—renewable energy, nuclear energy and green vehicles. Chen focuses on China's new energy industry as a key theme in China's narratives of its protection of human security. The development of this industry serves as an important aspect of China's somewhat unexpected rise into leadership in light of the unilateral withdrawal of the US from the global environmental governance under the Trump administration.

While there are continuities and consistencies with the pre-COVID policies, this chapter highlights the intensified contradictions between national security and human security during an international public health crisis. In its ambiguous 'Chinese-style' human security discourse, China adopts a rather limited view of human security, maintaining a firm grasp of what can and cannot be included in the human security discourse. Although Chen notes a shift towards 'people-based discussions', issues touching upon nationalism and human rights remain 'sensitive matters' which have been treated differently.

The new energy industry is an illustrative example of how state-led human security initiatives, championed by the National Security Commission, promoted the idea of 'non-state-centric security', the scope of which has been carefully managed within the broader discourse of 'building a harmonious society' in which the quality, as opposed to the rapid speed of development, has been brought back into focus. Large-scale crises like COVID-19 demonstrate the effectiveness of a capable central government in curbing the spread of the virus, and they also reveal that 'non-state' initiatives are eventually subordinated to a national security agenda, in which the priority of security concerns is determined by the state. Chen's discussion offers evidence for this observation by showing how environmental issues have taken a back seat during COVID-19 to allow the government to respond to the spread of the virus as well as the economic setback caused by it. As a result, the state's emphasis on the New Green Deal remains largely rhetorical. Essentially, this shift reveals the perception within the Chinese policy circles that the security of individuals as a result of the spread of the virus is more immediately and severely impacted than that of environmental precarity. Even before COVID-19, the insufficient energy supply in rural areas might present as a more acute challenge than environmental issues.

A continuity of China's alternative energy industry is the central role of the state. As the state defines and decides how to respond to non-traditional security threats, there is little room for bottom-up empowerment. Four decades have passed since the 1978 reforms, and central planning still plays an important role in incentivising or containing the growth of the new energy industry by giving or reducing subsidies. However, the prospect of human security discourse is not entirely hopeless. As the concept of human security enters public consciousness, what had been 'critical' becomes increasingly 'practical'—although the state does not necessarily engage in human security policies for the sake of individual human rights, the growing risk of disregarding human security makes it practically desirable to consider negative impacts on human security, even if the ultimate goal is but to ensure the legitimacy, thus the survival of the regime.

Complicating the contradictions between national security at the macrolevel and individual security at the microlevel, fragmented local governance adds an additional layer of analysis at the mesolevel. At the local level, negotiations among various local actors and interest groups slow down decision-making processes, which impedes the central government's efforts to protect the environment. The dynamics at the meso-level indicate that, even in China, where a strong central government is in firm control, the political and socio-economic realities cannot be reduced to a simple 'state vs. human' dichotomy. Between the state and individuals, local actors and interest groups engage in constant negotiations, which, sometimes unwittingly, put human security concerns on the table.

In 2020, China's state-led transition towards a green economy has given way to the measures to control the spread of COVID-19 and its economic setbacks. The effective nation-wide resource mobilisation was made possible by a temporary curtailment or suspension of the autonomy of the local governments. This changing central-local relationship captures the dynamics of China's transition towards a global environmentalist whereby the concept of human security is recuperated.

Chapter 5 looks at the impact of patriotic education in the post-pandemic Chinese state. This chapter demonstrates how the concept of human security is closely associated with the legitimacy of the CCP. The pandemic, first reported in Wuhan, has shaken the legitimacy and accountability of the CCP. Huang highlights how different the concept human security is in the Chinese context: while the CCP emphasises the idea of the security for the people, it avoids empowering individuals. The CCP's approach, therefore, underscores the need for an added layer of analysis: between the state and individuals, the security of the people as a collective is weighed more heavily than individual rights.

This emphasis on the collective is derived from a long-standing Confucian tradition and the CCP's memory of the 'humiliating' history of not being able to defend its sovereignty. The worry for the loss of national sovereignty has been effectively inscribed into the collective memory of the Chinese people through patriotic education. This rationale convinced the public that the security of the whole population, which can be made possible only by the CCP, should be the absolute prerequisite for the human security at the individual level. This rationale also means that the human security efforts look very different in China. Individual sacrifices were glorified and those who had suffered for the sake of the common good were set as models for others to follow, notable examples including the glorification of national heroes such as Lei Feng, Huang Jiguang and Qiu Shaoyun. The Chinese education system that places particular emphasis on unifying ideas is crucial for the aforementioned rationale to be instilled into the collective consciousness.

The impact of the COVID-19 on Chinese people has clearly gone beyond hindered access to food and resources. The widespread anti-China sentiments, exacerbated by politicians such as former President Donald Trump, have increased the mental vulnerabilities of the Chinese people. In response to this human security challenge, the CCP has relied on advancing nationalism, in this case, patriotic education, to boost its legitimacy.

This chapter explores a wide range of policy initiatives in the few years before, and during, the outbreak of COVID-19, as well as after schools reopened. Through first-hand sources such as photos and data from his fieldwork in Ningxia, Huang presents a detailed and vivid account of the intensity of patriotic education that rolled out in the name of the 'mental wellbeing' of students. The language of human security has been co-opted by the state to forge political loyalty, and necessary psychological interventions have been politicised to tackle the alleged 'ideological pollution' or 'mental contamination' that may threaten the regime.

Chapter 6 applies the concept of human security to examine transport-related social issues. The intersection of human security literature and transport literature generates some compound insights that have been under-explored in each discipline. In particular, Qiyang Liu focuses on the (im)mobility of lay-citizens as a social consequence of COVID-19 containment measures. Imposed and self-motivated immobility during the pandemic have given rise to human security concerns that otherwise have been thought to be resolved by China's rapid economic growth, for example, access to food and necessities during lockdowns.

Qiyang Liu examines the case of COVID-19 containment measures in Kunming, where imposed and self-motivated immobility are observed as a result of government regulations at different levels. A total of 186 families (519 residents) was interviewed, and 401 of 519 interviewees responded to the survey. Drawing on both qualitative and quantitative data, Qiyang Liu identifies six themes that undermine human security at the individual level: 'insecure access to food, insecure access to facemasks, insecure access to social activities, insecure access to social interactions, a lack of updated information about containment measures, and risk of infection due to outdoor activities'.

These findings once again highlight the paradox of China's human security programmes during the pandemic: containment measures have been relatively effective in containing the spread of the virus, thus protecting 'human' at the community/collective level, but the very measures to achieve this, as Liu demonstrates, have contributed to insecurities at the individual level. Frictions exist not only between the state and individuals, but also between the collective and individuals. The chapter depicts, in vivid detail, how the collective began to take on the role of policing to discipline individuals when the latter were unwilling or unable to observe containment rules. Considering the technical skills required to observe these rules, such as scanning health QR code, these rules were particularly unfriendly to the elderly. As a result, the elderly was excluded and denied mobility in the name of security of the collective.

Chapter 7 discusses how the measures that were designed to improve human security impacted negatively on individuals' mental health. Considering the extent to which China was able to enforce measures such as lockdown and social isolation, the case of China is particularly representative in demonstrating their negative effects. Compared to other earlier public health crises, measures against COVID-19 have been compounded by digital technologies. In this chapter, Zhang elaborates on how social media has exacerbated the psychological crises people were already experiencing.

Echoing Chapters 2 and 3, this chapter notes how the government's initial responses have resulted in negative emotional responses of the domestic public. Although Chinese online platforms are heavily censored, feelings of anxiety, sadness and anger quickly spread online. The censorship mechanisms, including the Great Firewall and blacklisting keywords, impede the free flow of information, creating an environment where misinformation can thrive. Fake news and conspiracy theories have led to panic buying, inviting more efforts on the part of the Chinese government to clear up rumours. At the same time, rumour-control is integrated into the censorship mechanisms, causing further confusion and grievances particularly when whistle-blowing is designated as spreading rumours. These mechanisms backfired and ignited widespread demonstrations when Li Wenliang, the whistle-blower reprimanded for spreading 'fake news' died on 7 February 2020.

Notwithstanding the role of social media in exacerbating mental health problems, it can be used for social support. It is also used by the authorities to deliver mental health services to the general public. Overall, this chapter highlights the controversies regarding the control of information: misinformation spreads more easily in digitised China and threats public order and social stability, but the government intervention and its monopoly in defining the 'rumour' may also cause grievances to fester.

Chapter 8 returns to the topics of the securitisation process of the pandemic as a public health emergency, which has been touched upon in a number of earlier chapters, though not necessarily using the language of securitisation. This chapter focuses specifically on China's legal and institutional structure of public health management and the process from 'a-securitisation' to 'hyper-securitisation', in which a clear shift in the authorities' approaches to the pandemic can be seen. Jia Liu's analysis of this process reveals that China's particular legal and institutional structure is conducive to delayed responses from the local governments.

A particular feature of Chinese legal and institutional structure this chapter introduces is the '*tiao-tiao/kuai-kuai*' system of a dual rule. '*Tiao*' and '*kuai*' indicates the direction in which policy diffusion takes place. The *tiao* approach emphasises policy-making drawing largely from expert knowledge—thus it reflects a vertical central-local bureaucratic structure, resembling a narrow piece that the Chinese word '*tiao*' refers to. The *kuai* approach emphasises the governance and coordination within a lower administrative level, as a result of the devolution of the governance of certain issues, as if they were dealt with as a 'lump' or 'block', which is the literal translation of *kuai*.

The initial chaos in the government's responses to the pandemic reveals the internal frictions of the fragmented system of *tiao-kuai*, as it is unclear who is to be responsible and who is to take the blame when things go wrong. The initial *kuai* approach disincentivised local government officials to address early warning of the pandemic and prevented timely responses. Later, when the central authority stepped in, the issue was quickly securitised, marked by Xi's launching of the 'people's war' against the virus—the 'invisible enemy' (Xinhua 2020) and the frequent declarations of 'wartime state'.

Jia Liu's efforts in clear up the ambiguity surrounding the translation of *anquan* resonate with Jones' discussion of the term. As *anquan* can be translated as both security and safety, the scope of securitisation is potentially broader in the Chinese context compared to Western contexts.

Hyper-securitisation has negative impacts on society as a whole. For example, the overuse of 'wartime state' has caused paranoia and fatigue. On the other hand, Jia Liu also highlights that the process of securitisation has played an important role in the Chinese context to overcome the bureaucratic hurdles in the *tiao-kuai* system. This further indicates that while tensions certainly exist between the state, society and individuals, human security at the individual level is not always in conflict with state and societal security, which opens up opportunities for further discussions on how to work *with* the government, rather than working *against* it, in order to achieve human security.

This chapter ends the edited volume with an optimistic note: in the context of the particular political and legal system in China, the interdependence of state and societal security and individual human security are forcing the government to give more substance to its rhetorical commitment to human security. In addition to external pressures in the form of international criticisms, sanctions and interventions, domestic pressures on the CCP to protect its citizens are becoming increasingly significant. As the survival of the regime is increasingly linked with human security at the community and individual levels, the concept of human security will hold increasing appeal in the Chinese context.

References

Albrecht, Ulrich, Christine Chinkin, Gemma Collantes Celador, Stefanie Flechtner, Marlies Glasius, Mary Kaldor, Kimmo Kiljunen, et al. 2007. 'A European Way of Security: The Madrid Report of the Human Security Study Group Comprising a Proposal and Background Report'. Madrid.

Breslin, Shaun 2015. 'Chinese Discourses of Human Security: Discursive Power and Defining the Terms of the Debate'. *Journal of Contemporary Asia* 45 (2): 243–65.

Callahan, William A. 2012. 'China's Strategic Futures: Debating the Post-American World Order'. *Asian Survey* 52 (4): 617–42. https://doi.org/10.1525/as.2012.52.4.617.

Chinkin, Christine, and Mary Kaldor. 2017. 'Second-Generation Human Security'. In *International Law and New Wars*, 479–526. Cambridge: Cambridge University Press. https://doi.org/10.1017/9781316759868.012.

Christie, Ryerson. 2014. 'The Siren Song of Human Security'. In *Routledge Handbook of Human Security*, edited by Mary Martin and Taylor Owen, 94–108. London; New York: Routledge.

Cui, Shunji. 2019. 'China in the Fight against the Ebola Crisis: Human Security Perspectives'. In *Human Security and Cross-Border Cooperation in East Asia, Security, Development and Human Rights in East Asia*, edited by Carolina G. Hernandez, Eun Mee Kim, Yoichi Mine, and Ren Xiao, 155–80. Security, Development and Human Rights in East Asia. Cham, Switzerland: Palgrave Macmillan.

De Larrinaga, Miguel, and Marc G. Doucet. 2008. 'Sovereign Power and the Biopolitics of Human Security'. *Security Dialogue* 39 (5): 517–37. https://doi.org/10.1177/0967010608096148.

Duffield, Mark. 2007. *Development, Security and Unending War: Governing the World of Peoples*. Cambridge: Polity.

Edkins, Jenny. 2008. 'Biopolitics, Communication and Global Governance'. *Review of International Studies* 34 (S1): 211–32. https://doi.org/10.1017/S0260210508007870.

Foot, Rosemary. 2011. 'The Responsibility to Protect (R2P) and Its Evolution: Beijing's Influence on Norm Creation in Humanitarian Areas'. *St Antony's International Review* 6 (2): 47–66.

Franceschet, Antonio. 2016. 'Global Legalism and Human Security'. In *A Decade of Human Security*, edited by Sandra J. MacLean, David R. Black, and Timothy M. Shaw, 31–38. London; New York: Routledge.

Gardiner, Michael E. 2009. 'The Grandchildren of Marx and Coca-Cola: Lefebvre, Utopia and the "Recuperation" of Everyday Life'. In *Globalization and Utopia: Critical Essays*, edited by P. Hayden and C. el-Ojeili, 220–36. Palgrave Macmillan UK. https://doi.org/10.1057/9780230233607.

Glück, Antje. 2015. 'De-Westernisation, Key Concept Paper.' Media Conflict and Democratisation.

Han, Li. 2000. 'Ubiquitous Threats: Questioning the Concept of the "New Security Concept" [无处不在的威胁—"新安全观"概念质疑]'. *World Economics and Politics* 10: 64–69.

He, Yilun. 2004. 'A Discussion on the National Security Outlook [国家安全观刍议]'. *Cass Journal of Political Science* 3: 117–24.

Hernandez, Carolina G., Eun Mee Kim, Yoichi Mine, and Ren Xiao. 2019. 'Human Security in East Asia: Beyond Crises'. In *Human Security and Cross-Border Cooperation in East Asia*, edited by Carolina G. Hernandez, Eun Mee Kim, Yoichi Mine, and Ren Xiao, 1–19. Security, Development and Human Rights in East Asia. Cham: Springer International Publishing. https://doi.org/10.1007/978-3-319-95240-6_1.

James, Paul. 2014. 'Human Security as a Left-Over of Military Security, or as Integral to the Human Condition'. In *Human Security and Japan's Triple Disaster*, edited by Paul Bacon and Christopher Hobson. London: Routledge.

Krause, Keith. 2014. 'Critical Perspectives on Human Security'. In *Routledge Handbook of Human Security*, edited by Mary Martin and Taylor Owen, 76–93. London; New York: Routledge.

Lefebvre, Henri. 2005. *Critique of Everyday Life: Vol. III*. London: Verso.

MacFarlane, S. Neil, and Yuen Foong Khong. 2006. *Human Security and the UN: A Critical History*. Indiana University Press.

Martin, Mary, and Mary Kaldor. 2009. *The European Union and Human Security: External Interventions and Missions*. London: Routledge.

Martin, Mary, and Taylor Owen. 2010. 'The Second Generation of Human Security: Lessons from the UN and EU Experience'. *International Affairs* 86 (1): 211–24. https://doi.org/10.1111/j.1468-2346.2010.00876.x.

———, eds. 2014. *Routledge Handbook of Human Security*. London; New York: Routledge.

Matlary, Janne Haaland. 2008. 'Much Ado about Little: The EU and Human Security'. *International Affairs (Royal Institute of International Affairs 1944–)* 84 (1): 131–43. https://www.jstor.org/stable/25144719.

Ministry of Foreign Affairs. 2002. 'China's Position Paper on the New Security Concept'. 31 July 2002. http://www.fmprc.gov.cn/mfa_eng/wjb_663304/zzjg_663340/gjs_665170/gjzzyhy_665174/2612_665212/2614_665216/t15319.shtml.

Newman, Edward. 2001. 'Human Security and Constructivism'. *International Studies Perspectives* 2 (3): 239–51. https://doi.org/10.1111/1528-3577.00055.

———. 2010. 'Critical Human Security Studies'. *Review of International Studies* 36: 77–94. https://doi.org/10.1017/S0260210509990519.

———. 2014. 'The United Nations and Human Security: Between Solidarism and Pluralism'. In *Routledge Handbook of Human Security*, edited by Mary Martin and Taylor Owen, 225–38. London; New York: Routledge.

———. 2016a. 'Human Security: Reconciling Critical Aspirations with Political 'realities''. *British Journal of Criminology* 56 (6): 1165–83.

———. 2016b. 'The Challenge of Human Security Policymaking'. In *New Approaches to Human Security in the Asia-Pacific: China, Japan and Australia*, edited by William T. Tow, David Walton, and Rikki Kersten, 213–23. Routledge.

———. 2017. 'Can Human Security Ideas Ever Be Truly "Critical"?' *European Journal of Human Security*, 27–38.

Nishikawa, Yukiko. 2010. 'Human Security in East Asia at a Turning Point'. In *Human Security in Southeast Asia*, 30–59. London; New York: Routledge.

Nordin, Astrid, and Lisa Richaud. 2014. 'Subverting Official Language and Discourse in China? Type River Crab for Harmony': *China Information*, March. https://doi.org/10.1177/0920203X14524687.

Paltiel, Jeremy T. 2011. 'Constructing Global Order with Chinese Characteristics: Yan Xuetong and the Pre-Qin Response to International Anarchy'. *The Chinese Journal of International Politics* 4 (4): 375–403. https://doi.org/10.1093/cjip/por017.

Ren, Xiao. 2019. 'Human Security in Practice: The Chinese Experience'. In *Human Security Norms in East Asia*, edited by Yoichi Mine, Oscar A. Gómez, and Ako Muto. Security, Development and Human Rights in East Asia. Cham, Switzerland: Palgrave Macmillan.

Sabi, Stella C., and Mark Rieker. 2017. 'The Role of Civil Society in Health Policy Making in South Africa: A Review of the Strategies Adopted by the Treatment Action Campaign'. *African Journal of AIDS Research* 16 (1): 57–64. https://doi.org/10.2989/16085906.2017.1296874.

Thayer, Carlyle A. 2000. 'China's "New Security Concept" and ASEAN'. *Comparative Connections: An E-Journal on East Asian Bilateral Relations* 2 (3): 65–75.

———. 2003. 'China's "New Security Concept" and Southeast Asia'. In *Asia-Pacific Security: Policy Challenges*, 89–107. Canberra: ANU Press.

'The Concept of Sustainable Security Is a Beacon That Illuminates World Peace [可持续安全观是照亮世界和平的一盏明灯]'. 2017. CPC News. 16 March 2017. http://theory.people.com.cn/n1/2017/0316/c40531-29148225.html.

Tow, William T., David Walton, and Rikki Kersten, eds. 2013. *New Approaches to Human Security in the Asia-Pacific: China, Japan and Australia*. London ; New York: Routledge.

UNDP. 1994. 'Human Development Report 1994: New Dimensions of Human Security'. 1994. http://hdr.undp.org/en/content/human-development-report-1994.

Wang, Xuan, Kasper Juffermans, and Caixia Du. 2016. 'Harmony as Language Policy in China: An Internet Perspective'. *Language Policy* 15 (3): 299–321. https://doi.org/10.1007/s10993-015-9374-y.

Wang, Yizhou. 2017. *Creative Involvement: A New Direction in China's Diplomacy*. London; New York: Routledge.

Wishnick, Elizabeth. 2010. 'Dilemmas of Securitization and Health Risk Management in the People's Republic of China: The Cases of SARS and Avian Influenza'. *Health Policy and Planning* 25 (6): 454–66. https://doi.org/10.1093/heapol/czq065.

Xi, Jinping. 2013. 'Follow the Trend of the Times and Promote World Peace and Development [顺应时代前进潮流 促进世界和平发展]'. 23 March 2013. http://cpc.people.com.cn/n/2013/0324/c64094-20893328.html.

———. 2014. 'Xi Jinping: Adhere to the Overall Security Outlook and Walking on the Road of Chinese National Security with Chinese Characteristics [习近平: 坚持总体国家安全观 走中国特色国家安全道路]'. Xinhuanet. 2014. http://news.xinhuanet.com/2014-04/15/c_1110253910.htm.

Xinhua. 2020. 'Xi Focus: Chronicle of Xi's Leadership in China's War against Coronavirus'. 7 September 2020. http://www.xinhuanet.com/english/2020-09/07/c_139349538.htm.

Yaqing, Qin. 2009. 'Relationality and Processual Construction: Bringing Chinese Ideas into International Relations Theory'. *Social Sciences in China* 30 (4): 5–20. https://doi.org/10.1080/02529200903342560.

Yu, Xiaofeng. 2018. 'Harmonism and the Construction and Possibility of General Security Theory [和合主义与广义安全论的建构与可能]'. *South China Quarterly* 1: 7–8.

Zhao, Tingyang. 2006. 'Rethinking Empire from a Chinese Concept "All-under-Heaven" (Tian-Xia, 天下)'. *Social Identities* 12 (1): 29–41. https://doi.org/10.1080/13504630600555559.

Zheng, Chen. 2016. 'China and the Responsibility to Protect'. *Journal of Contemporary China*. https://doi.org/10.1080/10670564.2016.1160500.

Zhong, Feiteng. 2015. 'Developmental Approach to Security: China's Grand Strategy [发展型安全: 中国的一项大战略]'. In *New Security Concepts and Construction of Security System [新安全观与新安全体系构建]*, edited by Yunling Zhang, 103–30. Social Sciences Academic Press.

CHAPTER 2

(Ir)responsible Centrality? External Representations of China's COVID-19 Diplomacy

Catherine Jones

Introduction

China's role in the COVID pandemic—as represented in Western Europe—has moved through different phases. First, China was the starting place of the virus. Second, China was viewed as the unfortunate location of a severe and deadly and as an authoritarian responder. Third, it was seen as the provider of protective equipment and contributor to the global response. Fourth, it has been seen as being unwilling to engage with the international investigation by the World Health Organisation (WHO). Fifth, it has been presented as embarking on 'vaccine diplomacy'.

In this chapter it is argued that these representations of China demonstrate the marked differences in state understandings of both 'human

C. Jones (✉)
University of St Andrew, St Andrews, UK
e-mail: cmj20@st-andrews.ac.uk

C. Zhang (ed.), *Human Security in China*,
https://doi.org/10.1007/978-981-16-4675-1_2

security' 'responsibility' between China and Western Europe. An undertone of these narratives is that China does not act as a 'responsible' state when assessed against criteria which are implicitly based on Western conceptions of human security and responsibility. In tandem with the emergence of this narrative of China as 'irresponsible', China has changed the audience of its narrative on COVID has changed through these phases. Following the rejection of China's assistance and criticism of both China's role at the outset of the pandemic (see for example, Brown and Wang 2020, 253; Ward 2020; Pavel and Engelke 2020; BBC 2020a) and reactions to some batches of personal protective equipment (PPE) during the escalation phase in Europe (BBC 2020b), along with reports that SinoVac is less effective than alternatives produced by companies based in the West (BBC 2021) (despite its approval by the WHO), China's focus with the vaccine has been in providing vaccine to developing states and neighbours, rather than engaging with more developed states (Mallapaty 2021). Why do these narratives matter? Fundamentally, they matter if 'something that is said about China resonates with an audience and gains popularity through repetition' (Breslin 2021, 227). In this sense inaccurate narratives that gain traction create a problem for China's international relations, especially in democratic states where public opinion will inform policy.

What does this tell us about China as a 'post-pandemic state'? First, this reinforces previous patterns of Chinese foreign policy behaviour, that it will try and constructively engage with Western powers, however, if Western powers choose to act in a destructive way, China will withdraw or focus on positive constructive engagements with other states around the world. Paradoxically, this may mean China increasingly engages with states that contribute to the negative narratives of China in Western states. Unlike the cautious and constrained China in the 1990s, Xi Jinping is not waiting for recognition or approval by Western states (Zeng 2020).

Second, China in a post-pandemic state will continue to follow a pragmatic approach to foreign policy rather than following an approach that is either conceptually designed or teleological. In an area like human security, China's pragmatism will see different aspects of the 'chocolate box' of human security concept take centre stage depending on the issue. Again, this is likely to feed narratives of 'irresponsibility' because it will continue to make China's policy preference difficult to predict and therefore also difficult to work alongside in seeking to achieve human security objectives.

China and Responsible Human Security

In the introduction of this volume, Zhang outlines distinct moments in the development of the human security concept and China's engagement with it. In this chapter she outlined that China's leaders have continued to expand approaches to 'human-centred' security through, for example, the New Security Concept and Ruan Zongze's (2012) critique of the Responsibility to Protect (R2P) and innovation of Responsible Protection. Domestically, there was the rise of phrases including 'putting the people first' (Ren and Li 2013, 34).

In the development of China's approach to human security it is also important to highlight the importance of health emergencies in driving forward this debate in China. After the SARS outbreak in 2003, China took major steps to create 'a better public health system for the protection of people's health, and decided to strengthen that system by significantly increasing public health measures related to the strengthening the prevention of major epidemics' (Ren and Li 2013, 32). In this respect, as Ren and Li point out 'The security of the people should entail the protection of people's wellbeing and the avoidance of threats of disease, hunger, unemployment, political oppression and/or environmental degradation' (2013, 35). Therefore, in order to achieve this objective, human security was predicated on the achievement of development. Ostensibly, this appears to position China's approach to people centred security closer to the Japanese approach to human security as 'freedom from want'.

This narrative of the evolution of the concept of human security in China indicates that rather than rejecting the concept as a potential threat to China, instead the Chinese government sought to engage and modify the contents of the concept. Between Western and Chinese approaches to human security and drawing on the definition from Newman in the Introduction:: '[i]n its broadest sense, "human security" seeks to place the individual – or people collectively – as the *referent* [emphasis in original] of security, rather than, although *not necessarily in opposition to* [emphasis added], institutions such as a territory and state sovereignty' (Edward 2001, 239). This need to define 'human' in the concept of human security, is echoed by Li and Yu, when they pose the question 'Does it ultimately apply to an individual, a specific group with (or even constituting) a sovereign entity or the whole human race?' (2013, 17). Here is the first central issue that is contentious between China and Western approaches—are we considering human as singular or a collective term?

The difference is whether it is more responsible to consider people individually or collectively in relation to security. I argue that Western approaches tend towards the individual and East Asian or Chinese approaches tend towards the collective (which in turn opens a greater debate on the level at which we should consider the 'collective'). In a critical review of the UN approach to human security by MacFarlane and Khoong they indicate that "… ultimately, the protection of communities rested in important measure with those communities themselves" (2006, 160). Similarly, Breslin (2015, 248) indicates, there has been a deliberate use of translation of 'human security', in his analysis he indicates the importance of this shift is in moving the understanding of 'human' from the lindividual to the collective. This approach opens up potential to consider human security on a scale with individuals at one end and collective action at the other, but there are a range of approaches in the middle.

In internal innovations in China, Zhang (introduction of this volume) outlines that there has been significant engagement with and unpacking of the term 'security' for example in 'developmental security' and the relationship between security, and stability. It is therefore necessary to unpack the differences in the usage of the term 'security', 'stability' and 'safety' in relation to how China understands and implements the concept.

In a 2015 review of the literature in China, Breslin teases out a further dynamic here, which is the evolution of safety as key determinant of security (2015, 256). In this paper, Breslin uses the 7 elements of human security from the UNDP report (1994) and outlines the places where the Chinese debates on human security have produced clear distinctions or where there are 'Chinese characterisitics'. In doing this he indicates that it is important to separate out both the level of analysis and the type of understanding of security that the Chinese discourse applies. In particular, in separating out these 7 elements (economic; political and societal; food; health; personal; ecological and environmental and community and cultural), health security with Chinese characteristics is: "(a) Relative safety from infectious diseases; (b) Access to adequate medical services." (Breslin 2015, 256). In relation to COVID-19 and China's domestic and international response we see both of these elements pursued through policy. Seeking to lockdown cities and households in order to seek to protect from the infectious disease, through the creation and distribution of vaccines, and in providing access to medical services through the rapid building of hospitals and provision of health supplies globally.

The second area of distinction is, therefore, in the narratives that emerged from the Chinese government and ministries was a concern with 'human safety' rather than human 'security'. What then is the difference between 'security' and 'safety' in understanding China's approach? This may be a minor distinction in English and indeed these terms are frequently used synonymously.

I argue that a key distinction between these terms is in the role of the state and the implications for state action. 'Safety' in English implying a degree of protection or being protected from a threat. Whereas security implies the absence of a threat, not necessarily implying the need for active protection. Breslin indicates 安全 (anquan) can be translated as both safety and security. His analysis of the Chinese discourses also indicates that the state is viewed as being the source of protection, rather than the source of the threat (Breslin 2015, 249). This view is supported by the Chinese discourse on human security fitting in with as being an element of development, as development is then understood to be state-centric. As a result, this enshrines the role of the state as a provider of safety against threats rather than providing a frame in which security can emerge.

This leads to another noteworthy element in the distinction in the Western approach of human protection versus human security. This is also not a new distinction. Indeed, it has been an international consideration since at least the creation of 'safe areas' in the context of the Bosnian conflict in the 1990s. Prior to the implementation of these safe areas there was a debate in the Security Council (UN resolution 819 of 16 April 1993) that these 'areas' should be protected, as former Ambassador Arria noted in original of the Spanish of the proposal rendered these as 'protected areas' however in the English and French translations this term was rendered as 'safe area', as Arria noted this arose partly because the term 'protected' was seen by some states as requiring active 'protection' (Jones 2019, Chapter 6). Notably the distinction between states on either side of the divide of the protection/safe seems to be reflected in subsequent debates on the Responsibility to Protect and also in Human Security.

The third noteworthy element of difference here is that China's approach has been strongly driven by an approach of 'learning from doing'. In the introduction of this volume, Zhang succinctly points out that China has adopted the phrase of human security, but not the content. Instead, developing China's own understanding of what human security is in China. Following Zhang's analysis, this indicates that China's approach is pragmatic in two senses: first, it is rhetorically pragmatic, allowing for China to agree with Western powers in terms of phrasing but mean something different in terms of practice; second, it is pragmatic in terms of implementation and trying not to focus on the objective and not the means.

The heart of Ruan's (2012, 29–30) critique of R2P was practical—how do you achieve the overall objective without making life substantially worse in the process? A similar practical critique has been consistent in China's statements in the UN Security Council, whereby, there is a consistent recognition that approaches to protection must be 'people-centred' but that must be reflected in the practice as well as the objective. Importantly, it should be noted that for China the entity doing the protecting is the state (although this may at times be fragmented in terms of the policymaking process) and therefore the state remains the central actor in protecting.

As a result of these significant points, I think it is instructive to consider the human security debate along two axes—the horizontal as being the understanding of 'human' as being on a continuum from individual to collective, and the vertical being from security to safety (or the agency of the state)—see Fig. 2.1.

A final important point here, is that although in Fig. 2.1, and in the narrative above I make the distinction between China and 'Western approaches' which may present a view that China's approach is unique or isolated from the rest of the international community, this is a misrepresentation. China's approach to collective human security rather than the individual level and the centrality of the state in providing a safe environment is shared by a number of states globally. Perhaps more significantly, it is important to note the variety within the grouping of 'Western' approaches, where difference also appears. Indeed, if we were to plot different state approaches along these two axes (at a single point in time—as these positions do change over time reflecting new challenges and experiences) we would see huge variety that exists in understanding this concept.

What then is 'responsible' in this schema of human security?

I argue this understanding of differences in understandings of the human security concept is also reflected in China's response to COVID-19. These

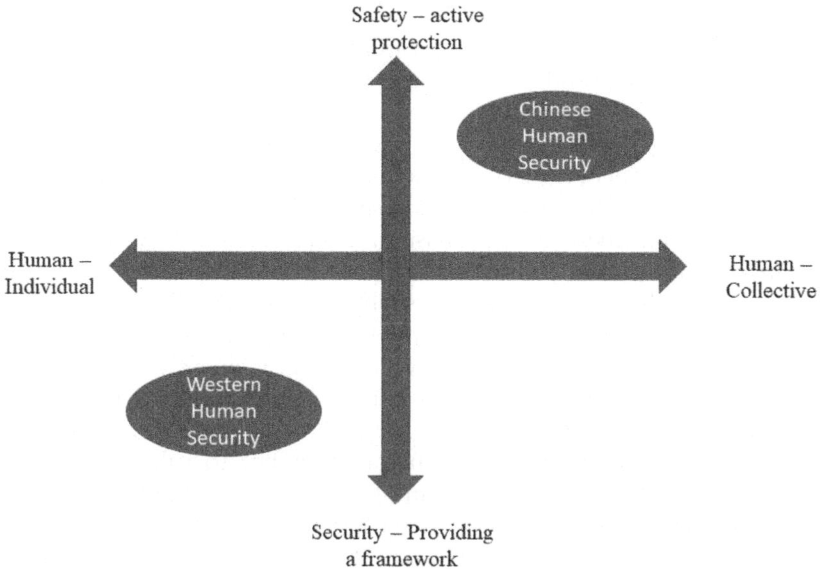

Fig. 2.1 Dimensions of human security (created by author)

differences then inform how states have acted, and also how they represent other states actions. In these representations it is also possible to see as informing the difference in understanding what is 'responsible' international behaviour in relation to COVID-19.

To be sure, debates about China and responsibility have been central in international relations in the twenty-first century. In 1995 on the sidelines of a UN meeting, the then President Bill Clinton welcomed China as a great power but also called on China to become a 'responsible great power' embedded within international institutions following the rules and norms set by those institutions (Hoo Tiang Boon 2018). Since then numerous scholars have engaged with the debate on whether China is a responsible great power: Xia Liping in 2010 made the argument that the integrated China becomes the more 'responsible' it will be; Breslin in 2010 considered China as a 'Dissatisfied responsible great power'; Yong Deng in 2014 claimed that China was a 'post-responsible great power'.

Running through all of these debates is an assumption that being responsible means either, conforming to the rules or norms, or (more specifically) conforming to the rules and norms as understood by Western powers. Nordin and Smith (2020) outline the importance in problematising the term 'responsibility'. They provide three different approaches in their analyses: (1) responsibility is following a set of rules or norms; (2) responsibility is a virtue 'concerned with the demands and burdens that being with other people places on us in terms of virtues, morals, or ethics beyond rules' (2020, no page); (3) responsibility is political 'a recognition of the unjustness of any decision. There are no solid foundations for making a decision about whose call for help is responded to, and in helping some there are always others who are not helped'.

These three approaches to conceptualising responsibility are central to the argument of this chapter. As noted above, Chinese understandings of human security have a different approach and emphasis to Western approaches, as such although adherence to either of these understandings may be seen as responsible in terms of adherence to rules and norms, both can represent adherence to an alternative understanding as being 'irresponsible'. It also provides us with a frame of analysis useful for assessing China's approach to COVID-19. In terms of the first element of the definition—adherence to rules and norms: this process is then more concerned with constructions of narratives of responsibility, rather than a straightforward assessment of compliance to rules and norms. As a result, we can set up our analysis to look at what China did and how it was represented in relation to the rules and norms. In the second approach to responsibility (as virtue) it is then important to consider the additional burdens or demands that a state might adhere to beyond the formal rules and norms. In the final element, I consider this in terms of the acceptance of legitimate boundaries—what a state knows is beyond their current capacity (this would connect to the Chinese critique of R2P that protection needs to improve on what exists rather than offer a potentially false hope).

Responsible Human Security and Covid 19—An Analytical Framework?
From the above discussions it is clear that in assessing China's approach to handling the pandemic both domestically and internationally a framework necessarily needs to reflect both different approaches to human security and different understandings of responsibility. And, in order to try and make a less pejorative assessment of China's actions, some clear criteria need to be presented in order to identify what China has done. This framework will enable us to accurately chart China's practice against these

definitions. In the final section of this chapter it will then be possible to explore how China has been externally represented and to compare these representations to the analysis of action (Table 2.1).

Table 2.1 Human security and responsibility (created by author)

		Approaches to responsibility		
		Upholding the status quo	*Virtue and ethics beyond the rules and burden taking*	*Recognising unjustness*
Approaches to human security	Individual—security	Focus on maintaining individual freedoms Creating a framework in which individual rights are protected	Providing a framework in which individual in other political authorities may be able to be safe (for example 'safe havens')	Acknowledging there are boundaries to who can be helped and where you cannot provide assistance
	Individual—safety	Seeking to maintain individual freedoms by providing for the protection of individuals	Seeking to maintain the freedoms for individuals in another political entity, through direct actions—for example through structural adjustment policies	
	Collective—security	Focus on protecting groups or communities, by providing a framework in which they can be secure	Seeking to provide framework for security for a group that may be outside your own legal requirements	
	Collective—safety	Focus on providing a specific set of obligations from a legal entity to a group or community—which may be at the expense of individual freedoms	Providing more that required for the safety of a particular community—focusing on provision for a wider number of communities that may be interconnected	

China, Human Security and COVID-19

On December 31, 2019, the World Health Organisation was made aware of a cluster of cases that were being understood as a new form of 'viral pneumonia'. According to the WHO timeline of events this was initially from a posting on the Wuhan Municipal health commission (WHO 2021a). On January 1, 2020 the WHO requested information on these cases, and on January 3 China provided information to the WHO. By January 30, 2020 the WHO declared this novel virus to be 'a public health emergency of international concern' (WHO 2021a). On March 11, 2020 the WHO declared the outbreak a pandemic.

Since the outbreak of the pandemic in China in late 2019, to May 2021 there have been an estimated 157 million cases, and over 3 million deaths (although these estimates are likely to be under the true number of those infected and deaths). Global responses have been mixed, (at time of writing) some states have been considered to have been highly successful in managing the outbreak (including New Zealand and South Korea) whereas other states have faced crises in managing the disease either in first or subsequent waves.

Reports of China's response have indicated that initially the PRC government may have sought to coverup the outbreak, but then acted decisively in imposing lockdowns of cities, travel restrictions, and rapidly constructing new hospitals to deal with the influx of cases. Initially this approach was viewed as 'autocratic and draconian' (Brown and Wang 2020, 254), however, as the disease spread and the capacity of health-care systems became stretched, even Western Liberal states imposed severe restrictions on individual liberties in order to stop the spread of the vaccine.

Despite evidence of the comparative success of China in some areas of responses to the outbreak including, managing the outbreak domestically, providing personal protective equipment (PPE) globally, and in developing a vaccine (SinoVac) and distributing vaccine to developing states, global narratives of China and COVID-19 have been overwhelmingly negative. In particular, President Trump referring to the virus as the 'China virus' on numerous occasions, and repeated claims that China tried to hide information from the WHO both when the virus was initially discovered, and during the subsequent WHO investigation into the origins of the virus.

Of these narratives Brown and Wang argue that 'A virus pandemic that originated from China therefore served as a metaphor for many of the other ills and problems that an audience anxious, and antagonistic to China's political and geopolitical nature, attributed to the new global actor' (2020, 254). This analysis points to the important connection between COVID-19 and China's actions to the broader debates in International Relations regarding China as a responsible power. As Breslin points out (2020) COVID has accelerated trends in understanding China as an assertive power.

At time of writing, the pandemic is still ongoing (May 2021) and it may take years to fully evaluate the states that have been successful or less successful and the efficacy of different specific policies. As a result, I will reserve judgement on proclaiming successes and failures at this stage. From the existing analyses, and these initial perspectives, Greer et al. (2020) propose a reasonable hypothesis:

> Authoritarian regimes are bad at maintaining the internal and external flow of good information, but only some are good at forceful action (Shih, 2020). The internal and external information flows of both China and Russia inhibited crucial information, but only China also chose and implemented really effective action. Democratic regimes might have more difficulty taking forceful or even appropriate action but can benefit from better information flow and public trust. (Greer et al. 2020, 1414)

From this hypothesis, one element stands out: democratic regimes have sought to protect the individual freedoms of citizens, at the expense of rapid and 'draconian' responses to the virus. Whereas China acted swiftly to impose constraints on individual liberties, in favour of protecting the collective of the state. This appears to being to reflect the different approaches to the understanding of 'human' in the conceptual discussion of human security above.

This brief overview points to the connection between COVID-19, and the conceptual discussion on human security and responsibility. They also indicate that China is central to global narratives and considerations of the future of geopolitics. The next two sub-sections will explore these two elements in more detail in relation to the framework above.

Representations of China's 'Responsibility' and COVID-19

International relations scholarship has long recognised the importance of representations in shaping relations between states and peoples. In a landmark text that considered representations of North Korea, Roland Blieker demonstrates the link between representations of North Korea and policy options:

> The inability to see political trends that contradict prevailing stereotypical images is linked to the overall representational practices that prevail in much of the Western world. Sigal demonstrates, for instance, that the United States often did not hear signs of compromise emanating from Pyongyang because the prevalent storyline about North Korea, one that revolves around an image of an aggressive communist state incapable of compromising, was simply too strong and deeply entrenched. (2005, xxxiii–xxxiv)

In the case of China and COVID-19 we have a clear example of the importance of how the framing of China throughout the pandemic appears to have shifted not only views of COVID-19, but also of whether China is a responsible power. In this section, I will present the narratives and how they have changed during the progress of the pandemic, increasingly highlighting that the negative frames of China's actions have had more resonance with Western publics. These negative frames are not only connected to COVID-19 but wider representations of how China views human security.

1. What is the status quo—setting a benchmark

Prior to the current pandemic of COVID-19, Western populations had largely been protected from outbreaks of a similar kind. The Ebola virus outbreak in 2014–2016 was centred on East Africa and the SARS outbreak in 2002–2004, was centred on East Asian states and originated in China. In both of these recent moments of epidemic Western states remained relatively isolated from infection and deaths.

In assessments of both of these cases the WHO and the United Nations have refined and developed their responses. Yet, in both cases the 'trigger' location took time to understand, identify and report the outbreak. In the case of Ebola, according to the summary from the Centre for Disease Control (CDC) in the United States, the first patient was identified in

December 2013, a medical alert was issued on January 24, 2014, on March 23, when the disease was present in the capital of Guinea Bissau, the government issued an alert for an 'unidentified illness' (CDC 2021). Only once the infection had spread to neighbouring states, did the WHO declare a public health emergency in August 2014.

In the SARS outbreak in 2002 the first potential case was identified in November 2002 and it was in March 2003 that the WHO issued an alert. At the time China was in a political dilemma, as Huang says 'it caused the most severe socio-political crisis for the Chinese leadership since the 1989 Tiananmen crackdown. Outbreak of the disease fueled fears among economists that China's economy was headed for a serious downturn. A fatal period of hesitation regarding information-sharing and action spawned anxiety, panic, and rumor-mongering across the country and undermined the government's efforts to create a milder image of itself in the international arena' (Huang 2004). Huang goes on to identify issues of data sharing were not restricted to China's openness with the international community but also internally within China. It was only in February 2003 that regional health officers from Guangdong spoke out about the disease (Huang 2004).

Following this outbreak, China was widely criticised for hiding information and not being open about a potential global threat. In Huang's (2004) analysis it is clear that not only were public health considerations important, but also all levels of government concerns over economic development and reputation were also important in determining whether to share information. This issue presented numerous problems for the government in China and once the infection rate was brought under control changes within China began to emerge. China became more engaged and open in sharing information internationally in relation to the range of other infectious diseases.

However, praise should also be slightly muted here as Sow Keat Tok notes (2013, 137–138), the need to effectively share information and work together on disease control did not spread to Taipei's application to become an observer member at the World Health Assembly (WHA) which later became the WHO. Which could indicate that political considerations also play a role in how China will respond to public health issues. Furthermore although the government in Beijing did make changes to internal governance related to the accurate reporting of potential outbreaks of disease, they also do not generate an expectation that the population should be informed. According to Huang (2004), 'Vice

Premier Wu Yi reiterated state control over the media in order to strictly prohibit the spread of rumors and other harmful information (Wu Yi 2003)'. Hence, on the one hand it is clear that China did tighten internal reporting structures following SARS, it also stunted public dissemination and sharing of information. In considering this in the best possible light, this could be seen as reflecting the view of human security outlined above, that the state has a clear role in protecting the population, and that includes avoiding the spread of potentially dangerous 'rumours'.

From these two epidemics in the twenty-first century it is clear that a common problem for health authorities is identifying what they are dealing with, and therefore what action is appropriate. Although, it would be helpful to compare the timelines for each outbreak from the first case to the declaration of an emergency, as all diseases are different it would be expected that the timelines would be different so this would not be a fair comparison. As a result, setting a clear benchmark for when reporting to the WHO should happen is more difficult. In the document on diseases surveillance published by the WHO there is a clear recognition of the need to develop internal reporting structures in countries that are resilient in the face of challenges of responding to an emergency, however the report also notes that this will vary between countries and they provide some assistance in terms of questions to consider in setting up these systems and documents that may be useful (WHO 2021b, 8).

So what is the 'status quo' in terms of expected reporting and standards? I argue that rapid reporting is essential however, what this looks like and when it happens will be determined by the state with the outbreak rather than the international community. However, the standards against which countries will be evaluated will be determined by the expectations, of the international community and these expectations will be a composite of both the WHO standards, their view of the capacity of the country and the spread of infection. Hence this benchmark is likely to be political as well as scientific, and therefore the representation of the country and the outbreak will be very important in determining whether the status quo has been upheld or not.

2. Did China challenge the status quo?

At the outbreak of the pandemic, in December 2019 and into January 2020, the pandemic was viewed and represented as being an issue for

China and the Chinese were working cooperatively (albeit with a delay) with the WHO. According to President Trump, before boarding Marine One on February 7, 2020, when asked if China was hiding the full extent of COVID-19:

> No. China is working very hard. Late last night, I had a very good talk with President Xi, and we talked about -- mostly about the coronavirus. They're working really hard, and I think they are doing a very professional job. They're in touch with World -- the World -- World Organization. CDC also. We're working together. (Factbase 2021; see also, Viala-Gaudefroy and Lindaman 2020)

In contrast in March 2020, Secretary of State Pompeo was briefing about the 'China virus'. However, according to the initial analysis from Viala-Gaudefroy and Lindaman (2020), President Trump's unfavourable briefings only emerged after the Chinese have promulgated the idea that the virus had been released in Wuhan by the US army.

In the UK the BBC was reporting the 'COVID 19: 5 days that shaped the outbreak', included in this report was a claim that China had evidence that there was a new virus but:

> International law stipulates that new infectious disease outbreaks of global concern be reported to the World Health Organization within 24 hours. But on 1 January the WHO still had not had official notification of the outbreak. The previous day, officials there had spotted the ProMed post and reports online, so they contacted China's National Health Commission. (BBC 2020a)

In a BBC documentary for the programme Panorama, Carrie Gracie also investigated the argument that China was hiding information on the outbreak of the virus. Other reports from the BBC have focused on the role of China's state media in covering up China's responses to COVID-19.

These two competing narratives present diametrically opposing views of whether China has acted responsibly in relation to the status quo. On the one hand, the BBC made clear that their reporters viewed that China was not conforming to the accepted approach and reporting the outbreak, on the other hand President Trump implied that the Chinese were actively engaged with the international community in managing the outbreak (see Brown and Wang, 2020).

As the pandemic progressed, reports about China that had a negative twist appeared to gain more resonance within western states. In March and April 2020 when the UK was facing tremendous challenges in providing personal protective equipment to hospitals and there were similar shortages across Europe, media reports highlighted the vast number of PPE imports from China (BBC 2020b). Despite this initial positive reporting, headlines focused on the few batches that were not adequate rather than the millions of pieces that were used to keep health workers safe. However, other reports emerged raising concern about China's 'dominance' over the PPE market and the benefits that Chinese firms get in setting up their operations (Bradsher 2020). Within this critique, it is clear that again despite the provision of supplies to a world in need, China was not being seen as conforming to the status quo, instead there was evidence that it was 'anti-competitive' in supporting these businesses.

Later in the crisis, it is also clear that China did not help itself. In attempting to investigate the origins of the outbreak Beijing's role in limiting the WHO researchers access both to enter China but also their access to relevant materials has potentially exacerbated the tensions and added fuel to fire of presentations that China is trying to hide something. As a result, although it may be possible to claim that during the initial outbreak in December 2019, China did act responsibly (albeit not in line with political expectations) in its subsequent engagement it has not acted responsibly in limited access to materials.

What effect do these narratives have? It would be easy to overstate the importance of this rhetoric and reporting. To be sure, prior to the Coronavirus, China was seen as being potentially irresponsible by Western states. However, according to polls by Pew and a Consortium of researchers at the Central Europe Centre for Asia studies, 'unfavourable' views of China have significantly increased in the year of the pandemic (Silver et al. 2021) noting that these views are related to understandings that 'China has handled the pandemic badly'. Is this to do with representations? According to an article in the Lancet (Burki 2021), China has handled the pandemic extremely well to date by controlling infections internally.

I argue that according to the framework—presented above—China's approach here has seemly been to share a burden (in respect to PPE) and has gone beyond the expectations in relation to providing support. Although in the first few days of the outbreak it may not have conformed to the expected speed with which other states would have liked China to report the outbreak, it did subsequently engage with the WHO and provided an ongoing stream of information regarding what had been successful in managing the outbreak. As a result, in relation to being 'responsible' it may be that China's action match a different understanding of what it means to be responsible.

Conclusion

From this probative study, it is clear that in its response to COVID-19, China has sought to provide human safety, to its own citizens considering the best for the community rather than the individual. This approach, which involves depriving people of liberty, but also imposing tracking of their movements on a national scale, has been seen as objectionable by the international community. Yet, despite their objectives, liberal democracies, including France, Italy and the UK have all had to impose temporary curtailments on liberties of individuals, however this is presented as a temporary aberration rather than a preference. This approach then seems to align China's practice with its conceptual view of human security as requiring action of the state in order to protect a collective group.

The second element that this study indicates is that China seeks to adopt a different approach to understanding what is responsibility. In some regards, China's action—particularly in supplying PPE and vaccines—goes beyond merely maintaining the status quo instead seeking to act to redress existing inequalities of the status quo. This does mean there is validity in the argument that China—as defined against the definition of maintaining the status quo—acts irresponsibly. However, there is increasing space to challenge that as the only definition of how to act responsibly. Finally, this chapter has indicated that China is represented as acting irresponsibly in relation to expectations of human security in Western narratives.

References

BBC. 2020a. 'Covid 19: Five days that shaped the outbreak' published January 26, 2020. Available https://www.bbc.co.uk/news/world-55756452 accessed 10 May 2021.

BBC. 2020b. 'Coronavirus: "NHS" passenger plane brings PPE from China' published on April 28, 2020. Available https://www.bbc.co.uk/news/uk-england-dorset-52460823 accessed 10 May 2021.

BBC. 2021. 'Sinovac: Brazil results show Chinese vaccine 50.4% effective' BBC, published January 13, 2021. Available https://www.bbc.co.uk/news/world-latin-america-55642648 accessed 12 May 2021.
Blieker, Roland. 2005. *Divided Korea*, University of Minnesota Press, Minneapolis, Minnesota.
Breslin, Shaun. 2010. China's emerging global role: Dissatisfied responsible great power. *Politics*, 30 (1_suppl), pp. 52–62. https://doi.org/10.1111/j.1467-9256.2010.01385.x.
Breslin, Shaun 2015. 'Chinese discourses of human security: Discursive power and defining the terms of the debate' *Journal of Contemporary Asia*, 45 (2), pp. 243–265.
Breslin, Shaun. 2020. Contribution to a roundtable November 2020, online.
Breslin, Shaun. 2021. *China Risen: Studying Chinese Global Power*, Bristol University Press, Bristol.
Brown, Kerry, and Ruby Congjiang Wang. 2020. 'Politics and science: The case of China and the Coronavirus' *Asian Affairs*, 51 (2), pp. 247–264. https://doi.org/10.1080/03068374.2020.1752567.
Burki, Talha. 2021. 'China's successful control of COVID 19' The Lancet. 8 October 2020. https://doi.org/10.1016/S1473-3099(20)30800-8.
CDC, 2021. *2014–2016 Ebola Outbreak in West Africa.* Avialable https://www.cdc.gov/vhf/ebola/history/2014-2016-outbreak/index.html accessed 13 September 2021.
Factbase. 2021. 'Press Gaggle: Donald Trump speaks to the Press before Marine One departure, February 7, 2020.' Available https://factba.se/transcript/donald-trump-press-gaggle-marine-one-departure-february-7-2020 accessed 10 May 2021.
Greer, Scott L., Elizabeth J. King, Elize Massard da Fonseca, and Andre Peralta-Santos. 2020. 'The comparative politics of COVID-19: The need to understand government responses' *Global Public Health*, 15 (9), pp. 1413–1416. https://doi.org/10.1080/17441692.2020.1783340.
Bradsher, Keith. 2020. 'China dominates medical supplies, in this outbreak and the next' *New York Times*, published July 5, 2020. Available https://www.nytimes.com/2020/07/05/business/china-medical-supplies.html accessed 10 May 2021.
Edward, Newman. 2001. Human security and constructivism. *International Studies Perspectives*, 2 (3), 239–251. https://doi.org/10.1111/1528-3577.00055.
Hoo Tiang Boon. 2018. *China's Global Identity: Considering the responsibilities of great power*, Georgetown University Press: Georgetown.
Huang, Yanzhong. 2004. 'The SARS epidemic and its aftermath in China: A political perspective' in Knobler S., Mahmoud A., Lemon S., et al., editors, *Learning from SARS: Preparing for the Next Disease Outbreak: Workshop*

Summary. Institute of Medicine (US) Forum on Microbial Threats, available https://www.ncbi.nlm.nih.gov/books/NBK92479/ accessed 13 May 2021.

Jia, Li, and Yu Xiaofeng. 2013. 'Human Security: China's conceptual approaches and policymaking patterns' in William Tow, David Walton and Rikki Kersten, *New Approaches to Human Security in the Asia-Pacific: China, Japan and Australia* (Rethinking Asia and International Relations) Ashgate, pp. 15–29.

Jones, Catherine. 2019. '*China's Challenge to Liberal Norms: The Durability of Liberal Order*' Palgrave Macmillan, Basingstoke.

MacFarlane, Neil S., and Yuen Foong Khong. 2006. *Human Security and the UN: A Critical History*, Indiana University Press, Bloomington Indiana.

Mallapaty, Smiriti. 2021. 'China's COVID vaccines are going global—but questions remain' *Nature*, published May 4, 2021, available https://www.nature.com/articles/d41586-021-01146-0 accessed 12 May 2021.

Nordin, Astrid HM and Graham M. Smith. 2020. China's Rise and "Responsibility" in the 21st Century. British Journal of Chinese Studies, 1040–1060. https://doi.org/10.51661/bjocs.v10i0.56

Pavel, Barry, and Peter Engelke. 2020. 'Irresponsible wet market practices led to COVID-19. China hasn't learned its lesson' *Euronews*, published 30 April 2020. Available https://www.euronews.com/2020/04/30/irresponsible-wet-market-practices-led-to-covid-19-china-hasn-t-learned-its-lesson-view accessed 12 May 2021.

Ren, Xiao, and Yanxing Li. 2013. 'A return to People: China's approach to human security' in William Tow, David Walton and Rikki Kersten, *New Approaches to Human Security in the Asia-Pacific: China, Japan and Australia* (Rethinking Asia and International Relations) Ashgate, pp. 31–42.

Silver, Laura, Kat Devlin, and Christine Huang. 2021. 'Unfavorable Views of China Reach Historic Highs in Many Countries' Pew Research Centre. https://www.pewresearch.org/global/2020/10/06/unfavorable-views-of-china-reach-historic-highs-in-many-countries/ accessed 10 May 2021.

Sow Keat Tok. 2013. *Managing China's Sovereignty in Hong Kong and Taiwan*, Palgrave Macmillan, Basingstoke.

UNDP. 1994. 'New dimensions of Human Security' in Human Development Report 1994 available http://hdr.undp.org/en/content/human-development-report-1994 accessed 12 May 2021.

Viala-Gaudefroy, Jerome, and Dana Lindaman. 2020. 'Donald Trump's 'China Virus' and the Politics of naming' The Conversation, published April 21, 2020 available https://theconversation.com/donald-trumps-chinese-virus-the-politics-of-naming-136796 accessed 10 May 2021.

Ward, Alex. 2020. 'How China is ruthlessly exploiting the coronavirus pandemic it helped cause' *VOX*, published 28 April 2020 available https://www.vox.com/2020/4/28/21234598/coronavirus-china-xi-jinping-foreign-policy accessed 12 May, 20201.

WHO, 2021a. 'Timeline: WHO's COVID-19 response' available https://www.who.int/emergencies/diseases/novel-coronavirus-2019/interactive-timeline#event-44 last accessed 8 May 2021.

WHO. 2021b. 'WHO recommended surveillance standards, Second edition' report number WHO/CDS/CSR/ISR/99.2 available https://www.who.int/csr/resources/publications/surveillance/WHO_CDS_CSR_ISR_99_2_EN/en/ accessed 13 May 2021.

Yong, Deng. 2015/2014. China: The post-responsible power. *The Washington Quarterly*, 37 (4), pp. 117–132. https://doi/org/10.1080/0163660X.2014.1002159.

Zeng, Jinghan. 2020. *Slogan Politics: Understanding Chinese Foreign Policy Concepts*, Palgrave Macmillan, Basingstoke.

Zongze, Ruan. 2012. 'Responsible protection: Building safer world' *China International Studies*, 34, pp. 19–41.

CHAPTER 3

Human Security and the Party-State-Society Triangle: Rethinking the CCP's Legitimacy Management in COVID-19

Hai Guo

Introduction

In December 2019, COVID-19, an infectious respiratory illness caused by a newly discovered coronavirus called SARS-CoV-2, was found in Wuhan, the most populous city in central China. In less than a few months, COVID-19 spread across continents and the world was precipitated into a global pandemic. Why was the Wuhan government slow to publicize the discovery of COVID-19 in December 2019? Was the initial failure on the part of the Wuhan government to inform the Chinese public about COVID-19 attributable to China's political system? Did the CCP experience legitimacy deficits because of the initial mishandling of the coronavirus? How did the CCP overcome the legitimacy crisis?

H. Guo (✉)
Institute of Public Policy (IPP), South China University of Technology, Guangzhou, China
e-mail: guohai@scut.edu.cn

C. Zhang (ed.), *Human Security in China*,
https://doi.org/10.1007/978-981-16-4675-1_3

Overall, what does the COVID-19 crisis tell us about the CCP's legitimacy management? In this chapter, I will address these questions with reference to human security and literatures on the CCP's legitimacy. Addressing these questions is crucial to the studies of Chinese politics for two reasons.

First, in so far as the provision of health security remains a vital source from which modern states draw legitimacy, loyalty and support from their citizens, the CCP must adapt to the changing standard and conceptualization of health and hygiene, or, to quote Michael Foucault, 'to ensure, sustain, and multiply life, to put this life in order' (Foucault 1990, 138). The association between hygiene and modernity implies that health security has become increasingly crucial to the Chinese ruling elites' legitimacy. As Rogaski (2004) reminds us, the meaning of hygiene is fluid, changing over time under different societal contexts. During the Republican era of 1912–1949, hygiene signified a desire for modernity—a collective consciousness that has since then persisted in the Chinese mindset. Health security became especially salient in the wake of the dissolution of the Soviet Union, which transformed the grand narrative of international politics from an ideological struggle between Capitalism and Communism into an economy-oriented struggle for development and modernization, in which health of individuals occupies a central position. The concept of 'human security' was introduced by the UNDP in 1994. It signalled a shift of post-Cold War security paradigm away from physical integrity of the state toward biological integrity of the individual.

Second, the COVID-19 pandemic, unprecedented as it is, is not the first public health crisis that put the performance of China's political system into test. In the early years of the PRC's foundation, the central government of China coordinated a nationwide campaign, the Patriotic Hygiene Movement, in attempts to put in place a 'great leap-forward' of hygiene level in the rural area. Apart from exterminating germs and pests, the campaign purported to construct a new image of the socialist state as clean and modern. More recently, in 2003, the SARS crisis became yet another benchmark against which the Party's performance was measured, as the epidemic exposed the weaknesses of China's national health system in a risk society, and, more importantly, the bureaucratic inertia that led to the irresponsiveness to the epidemic in the first place (Freedman 2005). Despite severe censorship, China's attempt to maintain secrecy at the early stage of the SARS outbreak has become, domestically and internationally, a constant source of criticisms against the efficiency, if not legitimacy of China's political system.

Just as how China's response to the SARS crisis of 2003 informed scholarly enquiries into the relationship between crisis and governance (see: Thornton 2009; Wishnick 2010; Chan et al. 2012), analysing China's response to the COVID-19 pandemic can reasonably sharpen our perception of the relationship between state legitimation process and human security. As good health is 'both essential and instrumental to human survival, livelihood and dignity' (Human Security Unit 2013, 27), public health security is widely considered an indispensable part of human security. The issue is particularly significant to the CCP, whose political legitimacy has rested, as Zhao Dingxin (2009) argues, upon performance rather than democratic procedure. Providing citizens with human security against infectious diseases, thus, has become a political mission for the CCP. Infectious diseases can put as much strain on China's public health system as on the Party's leadership.

My argument to the questions raised in this chapter is two-folded: (1) The CCP suffered from a legitimacy deficit on the eve of the COVID-19 outbreak in Wuhan, but it managed to overcome the legitimacy crisis. (2) Both the deficit and the subsequent recovery of the CCP's legitimacy were attributable to a unique feature of China's political system, or what I term the 'party-state-society triangle'. Here, I use the concept of 'party-state-society triangle' as a heuristic device to demonstrate how China's political system is conducive to, but simultaneously capable of overcoming, such massive human security crisis as COVID-19.

I will now turn to examine how the pandemic was generated by the party-state-society triangle. And then, I will look at how the party-state-society triangle enabled the CCP to overcome the legitimacy crisis, before engaging in a more theoretical discussion on the CCP's legitimation process with reference to scholarships relevant to the subject of the CCP's political legitimacy in China study.

The Party-State-Society Triangle and Public Health Crisis

The Party-State-Society Triangle

The party-state-society triangle refers to the power relationship between the central authority (the CCP and its core leadership), the local authority (the bureaucrats and state cadres at provincial, municipal, or township level), and the society. The party-state-society triangle is characterized by a powerful central authority that obstructs direct social transactions between the local authority and the society. On the one hand, the central authority commands the evaluation system of the local state cadres; on the other hand, it controls the society's freedom of speech. As a result, the relationship between the local authority and the society is marked by tensions and a lack of mutual trust: The local authority lacks the incentive to bargain and develop organic relationships with the society; the society tends to have a deep-seated distrust toward the corrupted local authority while it expects intervention from the central authority. In this context, popular distrust of the local authority became a useful asset, rather than a deficit, for the central authority: In situations of social instability or crises, the central authority intervened on behalf of the society to discipline the local authority, thereby rebuilding its political hegemony vis-à-vis the society. I argue that this process explains how the CCP/the central authority has been able to legitimate itself without electoral democracy. Just as how a father can derive love from his children by playing with the relationship between his children and their mother, the central authority can derive legitimacy by triangulating the tensions between the local authority and the society.

The party-state-society triangle functions differently in times of normal politics from it does in times of crises. In times of normal politics, the party-state-society triangle is conductive to crises; but in times of crises, it enables the central government to respond to the crisis efficiently. The party-state-society triangle is conducive to crises, because the power dynamics of the party-state-society triangular dictates that state cadres are accountable only to their superior rather than the public. As the local authority has little motivation to consider public accountability and transparency, over time, the societal system accumulates risks and thereby becomes susceptible to crises of human security, such as outbreaks of infectious diseases. However, the central government is able to respond to crises efficiently, because its monopoly on the state cadre evaluation and the society's freedom of expression allowed it to whip cadres, with reward and punishment, into large, campaign-style mobilization against public health crises, attribute wrongdoings to local cadres, and manage resources in unnegotiable terms.

When the COVID-19 was initially discovered in Wuhan, the party-state-society triangle worked against a good information flow between the Wuhan local authority and the public, and led to the outbreak of the pandemic. But when the pandemic emerged, the party-state-society triangle allowed the central authority to impute blames to the local state cadres, present itself as a benign, paternalistic arbiter, and claim the leadership to mobilize the whole society against the pandemic, hence preserving its political legitimacy and improving controls over the state apparatus. In other words, the CCP legitimated itself by solving crises that are created by the very system over which it commands authority.

The Party-State-Society Triangle as an Institutional Cause of the COVID-19 Outbreak in Wuhan

The party-state-society triangle, as a power relationship, is reproductive of what Zhou Xueguang terms the 'upward accountability system', a behavioural pattern in the Chinese bureaucracy 'in which officials are evaluated, rewarded, and allocated through a top-down process' (Zhou 2020, 479). Such a system is effective for implementing top-down orders, but inductive to the obstruction of information flow from the bottom up. As promotions and punishments are made, almost entirely, on the basis of the cadre evaluation system, local officials adhere steadfastly to orders from the top and, meanwhile, they are just as strongly motivated to mispresent and distort local information, especially in light of events deemed unfavourable to their evaluation. Human security is, therefore, often considered expendable and secondary to political considerations.

This does not mean that local officials are inefficient in dealing with crises of human security. In the initial discovery of COVID-19, local officials made more efforts than outsiders imagined to address the problem. What the upward accountability system led to however, was the predilection on the part of local officials for solving problems on their own, instead of reporting them to the upper level. When cadres share information in conformity to an institutionalized framework from the bottom up, they are often seen as shouldering off their responsibilities. Thus, information-sharing tends to result in negative performance evaluation, and even punishment of local officials. In particular, a cadre who reports each instance of emergency to the top is usually perceived by their superiors as inept (Zhou 2012, 112). Therefore, consideration for performance evaluation often outweighs the obligation to follow protocols. When a crisis of human security occurs, local authorities prefer handling the problem through informal channels to circumvent the institutional mechanism, in order to avoid getting on the nerves of their leaders. So in practice, the party-state-society triangle is translated into not simple bureaucratic inertia, but the suspension of formal institutional system in support of information sharing.

The party-state-society, as a heuristic device, can lend us insights into what happened in Wuhan on the eve of the COVID-19 outbreak between December 2019 and January 2020. Although the local government of Wuhan—along with health agencies including the Wuhan Municipal Health Commission (WMHC) and the local hospitals—knew of the existence of a then SARS-like pneumonia in as early as December 2019, they circumvented the web-based reporting system in attempts to confine the crisis-management process to the municipal level.

Safe Until Proven Infectious?

The earliest patient of the coronavirus remains unknown.[1] What can be confirmed thus far is that Wuhan is where the virus was first detected. As early as November 2019, there were on average one to five cases reported to hospitals in Wuhan each day (Davidson 2020). As hospitals in Wuhan began to receive an increasing number of patients with lung diseases with SARS-like symptoms, fear of the outbreak of a SARS-like epidemic started to spread among medical workers.

On 31 December 2019, the WMHC issued 'urgent notices' to city hospitals and the World Health Organization (WHO) regarding cases of Pneumonia of Unknown Etiology (PUE) in connection to the city's Huanan Seafood Wholesale Market. This announcement marked the official day that COVID-19 began to draw official and international attention. Despite the urgent notice, by late December 2019, it remained unconfirmed whether COVID-19—then still a scientifically understudied virus—was human-to-human transmissible. Two government documents, which were leaked to the public, said that 'pneumonia with unknown origin appeared in Huanan Seafood Market in Wuhan' (Zhao 2019). However, the WMHC, in an official announcement on 31 December

[1] Some sources suggest that the 'patient zero' can be traced back to November 2019, when a 55 year-old from Hubei province was suspected to have been diagnosed as infected with a SARS-like virus.

2019, claimed that 'there is so far no evidence that the virus is human-to-human transmissible' and that 'no medical staff has been infected with the virus' (WMHC 2019).

Human security was not given sufficient attention by the local authority of Wuhan at the initial stage of the pandemic, as the local officials played down, if not underestimated, the contagiousness of COVID-19. On 31 December, the WMHC said it had not yet informed the public about the virus, though it did establish an emergency task force to investigate 'the possibility of an epidemic' (*Caixin*, 31 December 2019). But regarding when they established, and who were members of, the task force, the WMHC replied that 'it needed to wait for official notice' (ibid.). Notwithstanding the 27 confirmed PUE cases—7 of them in critical condition and 2 returned to their community—the municipal government's attitude towards the SARS-like virus displayed more certainty than caution, so much so that COVID-19 appeared to be safe until proven infectious. On 31 December 2019, a bulletin on the WMHC official website stated that 'no human-to-human transmission has been detected' and that 'the disease is preventable and controllable' (*Caixin*, 31 December 2019). The reassuring tone was orchestrated by *People's Daily*, which, in a Weibo post on the same day, proclaimed that even if SARS reappeared, the country should be able to contain it with their 'robust disease prevention and control system' (ibid.).

The Absence of the Web-Based Reporting System

The 'robust disease prevention and control system' to which *Renmin Ribao* referred is the China Information System for Disease Control and Prevention (CISDCP), a nationally standardized network-based infectious disease reporting system, developed in the aftermath of SARS in 2004. Coordinated by the Chinese Center for Disease Control and Prevention (China CDC), the CISDCP serves, with 'a web-based, real-time reports covering 37 diseases across all areas of the country' (Wang et al. 2013), to empower the Chinese health system with 'unprecedented ability to detect, analyse, prevent, and respond to any communicable disease outbreak in the country' (ibid.). The system was a technological solution to the organizational problem of bureaucratic fragmentation, e.g. the lack of vertical and horizontal coordination of the Chinese health system in reporting and organizing effective measures to contain infectious diseases—a problem proved fatal in the SARS crisis of 2003. With the CISDCP, medical staff could directly report individual cases of infectious diseases online, reducing reporting time from 5 days to 4 hours (Wang et al. 2017).

But the technologically advanced infectious disease surveillance system was not put into operation to detect PUEs until 24 January 2021, the 28th day into the coronavirus outbreak. The first publicized report of COVID-19 as PUE appeared on 27 December 2019, when the Hubei Provincial Hospital of Integrated Chinese and Western Medicine reported 7 cases of 'unknown lung disease' to the Wuhan Jianghan Centre for Disease Prevention and Control. Zhang Jixian, who, with acute professional instinct, noticed the possible emergence of a SARS-like pneumonia. She reported the PUE to the local authority on 26 December 2019 (Xinhuanet 2020). Zhang's report was then directed, successively, to the Infection Control Department, the Medical Department, and the Hospital Director. Experts of the hospital were summoned to a meeting on the cases reported, and, afterwards, the deputy director of the hospital decided to report the PUE cases to the infectious disease control department of, respectively, the Wuhan Municipal Health Commission and the Hubei Provincial Health Commission (Tian and Chen 2020).

What is striking about the process above is the complete absence of the advanced web-based report system, which was installed nationwide to overcome the problem of bureaucratic fragmentation impeding effective and quick responses to the emergence of PUEs. According to 'National Scheme on the Detection, Inspection, and Management of Pneumonia of Unknown Etiology' as issued by the National Health Commission, medical staff in any hospital across the country is obliged, upon the detection of any PUE, to upload reports via the CISDCP within 12 hours (NHC 2007). However, Zhang's report on the novel coronavirus, instead of being documented upwardly to the national health department or the web-based reporting system, was initially circulated within the hospital and health commissions at the municipal level.

When Zhang Jijiang was asked by a journalist whether she had filed the report via the CISDCP, she replied that she simply did not know of it and was too preoccupied with treating patients to get her hands on it (*The Paper* 2020). Zhang's account must be taken with a pinch of salt. The China CDC has engaged consistently in training medical staff across the nation to operate the CISDCP for more than a decade, and there is little evidence that the web-based system was not in a routine operation. Six months before the coronavirus outbreak, Head of the Chinese CDC, Gao Fu, was cited as touting, in a Boao Forum for Asia in June 2019, how the CISDCP reassured ad augmented the robustness of China's public health system: 'We have a nation-wide system that covers every corner of our country. Any outbreak of epidemic would be notified to the health department within 6 hours' (Wang et al. 2020a). Even if Zhang Jijiang were unfamiliar with the protocol, other medical workers of the hospital should have been aware of and reported PUEs via the web-based reporting system. But that did not happen.

An alternative and more plausible account to explain the absence of the web-based system in reporting COVID-19 is that the medical staff of the Hubei Provincial Hospital of Integrated Chinese and Western Medicine were attempting to deal with the virus without using the CISDCP. They saw using the CISDCP as a risk, and their risk-averse tendency was conditioned by the Chinese bureaucratic culture, which is widely observed throughout hospitals in China. For instance, a research on how doctors reported PUEs in two top-tier hospitals in Anhui province in 2016 shows that only 1 out 335 PUE cases were processed via the web-based reporting system (Wang et al. 2017). This resulted from the discrepancy between the protocol that frontline medical workers were told to follow in theory and the limited resources they had at their disposal in dealing with public health emergencies in practice (ibid., 431). Physicians who followed the formal protocol to file a report via CISDCP might well find themselves being pushed into the awkward position of having to shoulder, and making their leaders assume, the responsibility of bumping up the hospital's workload and wasting medical resources. Therefore, it is one thing to follow the protocol, but quite another to assume responsibilities for sounding the alarm. The organizational feature of the Chinese bureaucracy made hospitals more inclined to circumvent rather than to share information in the face of an unknown infectious disease. In other words, the party-state-society triangle was still at work to impede the flow of information regarding PUEs between hospitals and CDCs despite the operational availability of a technologically superior surveillance system.

The way the WMHC handled PUE cases in early January 2020 is a case in point. On 3 January 2020, doctors from the Public Health Department of the Central Hospital of Wuhan enquired the Wuhan Jianghan Center For Diseases Prevention and Control about the treatment of 7 PUE cases. But the latter replied that they had to 'wait for instruction from the upper-level department' (*The Paper* 2020). It was not until 8 January that the Central Hospital of Wuhan managed to report 14

PUE cases to the WMHC. But even when the PUE cases were publicized locally, the leaders of the WMHC instructed that any PUE case, before being reported to China CDC, must be cascaded through the district, the municipal, and the provincial CDCs (Fan 2020). This instruction put in place an overly high diagnostic standard, precluding early reporting of PUE cases to the upper-level department. To prevent their medical workers from publicizing the coronavirus, the hospital administration of the Central Hospital of Wuhan went so far as to proscribe the use of vital medical equipment such as masks, goggles, and protective coveralls in several departments (ibid.). A doctor was even reprimanded by the hospital administration for wearing a mask in a meeting, for doing so might alarm the public of the fact that the hospital was taking precautionary measures against potential outbreak of an infectious disease (ibid.). Such proscription, which was made entirely on political consideration, led eventually to the tragic death of three doctors in the ophthalmology department.

If the doctors themselves were impelled by their professional ethics to inform the public about the PUE, their impulse would be suppressed by the local authority, which prioritized social stability over human security. Severe censorships were imposed upon doctors, forbidding private communications among them on WeChat about pandemics and pneumonia, or any keyword that can be dimly interpreted by the authority, or the AI, as detrimental to social stability (Crete-Nishihata et al. 2020). On 31 December, eight doctors who discussed with their colleagues about COVID-19 in their private WeChat group were reprimanded by the local police for 'spreading rumours'.

Even though the news about COVID-19 in Wuhan had gone public and international between 3 and 14 January 2020, Wuhan's local authority continued to be equivocal on the contagiousness of the virus. The WMHC, by 5 January, acknowledged the detection of PUE cases, but insisted that 'no tangible evidence of human-to-human transmissibility has been found' (WMHC 2020a). By 13 January, the day when the death of a patient with the COVID-19 in a Wuhan hospital was reported and a Chinese tourist from Wuhan was diagnosed in Thailand as infected with the coronavirus, the WMHC remained reserved, if not optimistic, about whether the virus was human-to-human transmissible, insisting that they 'cannot rule out risks of human-to-human transmissibility, but such risks remain low' (WMHC 2020b). The lack of clarity on the contagiousness of the COVID-19 was reinforced by the Beijing-based respiratory expert Wang Guangfa, who, on 11 January, said that the epidemic was 'preventable and controllable' (Liao and Li 2020). Such liberal assessment regarding the contagiousness of the virus continued to be upheld into the mid-January. On 19 January, the Director of Wuhan Municipal Health Commission Wang Gang said in a news conference: 'our initial impression is that the contagiousness of the epidemic is not very severe...With the implementation of prevention and control measures, the epidemic is preventable and controllable' (Liao and Le 2020).

20 January marked the turning point of China's response to the COVID-19 pandemic. On that day, Zhong Nanshan, a doctor heralded as a hero in the SARS crisis, stressed in a television interview that 'the coronavirus is for sure human-to-human transmissible' (*Renmin Ribao* 2020a). Zhong Nanshan's comment contrasted against the cautiousness of the WMHC and aroused a deluge of critical discussions in the public. Soon, the Internet was amassed with criticisms pointing to the concealing of coronavirus-related information from citizens by the Wuhan local authority. On 27 January, under intense public anger, Wuhan Mayor Zhou Xianwang, in a television broadcast, admitted the lack of information disclosure to the public at the early stage of the epidemic. While acknowledging the 'untimely information disclosure', the Wuhan mayor complained that 'as local authority, we can only disclose information after being authorized. This is not understood [by the public] at that time' (Caixin 2020).

The mayor's self-justification points to a historically persisting power dynamics between the local authority and the central authority in Chinese politics. In the Mao era, the distortion of local information was one of the major causes of the human disasters during the Great Leap Forward between 1958 and 1960. Local state cadres were pressured by their political superiors into reporting falsely inflated figures of grain and steel production (See: Bachman and Bachman 2006), and they kept silent about the prevalent starvation across the rural area, even in the face of cannibalism taking place, for fear of being accused of the crime of 'counter revolution' (Wemheuer 2010, 189).

Although China's political system in the post-Mao period is marked by de-centralization and bureaucratic fragmentation (Hameiri and Jones 2016), the relationship between the central authority, the local authority, and the society remained almost intact. The central authority still exercised absolute control over the cadre evaluation system; moreover, it found the cadre evaluation system an increasingly useful instrument of social intervention (see: Whiting 2017). Under the cadre evaluation system, local state cadres often find themselves caught in a dilemma. First, they need to be cautious not to trespass their leaders' authority. Humility—that is, not taking their leaders' credit—is considered a crucial 'merit' of a 'good cadre'. To demonstrate this 'merit', a 'good cadre' withholds from taking initiations seen as deviating from the normal routine, unless authorized by their leaders to do so. Second, the desire for reward, combined with the fear of punishment, compels cadres to misp-resent or distort local information, often at the expense of public interests and health security.

Considering that hospitals in Wuhan have been already equipped with an advanced web-based reporting system, the lack of information-sharing in December 2019 was unlikely an issue of technicality. Rather, it is better accounted for as a result of the conscious attempt by local cadres of the Wuhan health system to set up a bureaucratic barricade, with the design of circumventing the web-based reporting system and cautioning medical staff against passing on PUE-related information up to the national level authority or down to the public. On the one hand, in the face of a then scientifically unknown virus, the municipal authorities, without any clear authorization from the top, were making decisions in a mist, fearing that they might have to assume the responsibility of setting off a 'false alarm'. Moreover, on the consideration of festive events, local economy, and the then upcoming political meetings, the local bureaucrats of the Wuhan public health system were more incentivized to draw out the risk of accountability than to make evidence-based decisions in the interest of the public health security (Zhang et al. 2020). The actions that led to the protracted information flow in Wuhan was not a result of individual misbehaviours (e.g. not knowing how to use the web-based reporting system); instead, it was the systemic effect of China's bureaucratic culture as characterized by the party-state-society triangle.

The Party-State-Society Triangle and the CCP's Legitimacy Management in COVID-19

Attribution of Responsibilities, Management of Social Opinions, and Mobilization Against the Virus

In time of normal politics, the party-state-society triangle is conducive to crises; but in time of crises, it becomes a solution. Through the 'party-state-society triangle', the CCP aroused within the society a fantasy for a benign patriarch, who stepped in on behalf of the society to punish the corrupted local authority, restoring chaos back to order. We may consider the party-state-society triangle as having three concurring sub-processes: first, the attribution of responsibilities to the local authority; second, the management of social opinions; and third, draconic mobilization against the public health crisis. These sub-processes jointly redirected public sentiment onto local state cadres, who were dramatically scapegoated, and, in turn, framed the central authority as a reliable provider of human security for the society.

Attribution of responsibilities. As Thorton observes, public health crises are not natural occurrences, but socially constructed narratives that 'involve attributions of blame and proposed solutions' (Thornton 2009, 47). After China entered into a national emergency from 20 January 2020 onwards, a 'fast-track-dismissal' process kicked in to put a lid on the simmering public anger. First, the central government framed itself as a disciplined arbiter intervening in disputes between the society and the corrupted local government. The process started with the propagation, well-choreographed by the state-run media, of Xi Jinping's leadership in responding to the pandemic. Xi Jinping declared the imposition of an unprecedented city-wide lockdown upon Wuhan on 22 January 2020, commanded on 27 January all party members to implement containment measures in conformity to the central authority's order (The State Council Information Office of the People's Republic of China 2020, 16), and, on the next day, met with WHO Director-General Tedros Adhanom Ghebreyesus in Beijing to promulgate China's readiness to engage with the international community on preventing and controlling the pandemic. In addition to inducing public confidence with a positive image of an proactive national leader, Xi Jinping distanced himself from the local government. On 3 February Xi Jinping published an article on *Qiushi*, the party's leading theoretical journal, in which he claimed that he had, *as early as in a previous meeting of Politburo Standing Committee held on 7 January*, instructed on the prevention and control of the coronavirus in Wuhan (Xi 2020a). It means that Xi Jinping had ordered the top echelon of the communist party to tackle to pandemic almost two weeks well before the official announcement that the outbreak of the coronavirus was human-to-human transmissible. This gave the public a fair enough intimation that Xi 'has done his part'.

Meanwhile, a great number of local officials, especially in Wuhan, were purged by the central authority to demonstrate the government's public accountability. On 28 January 2020, the Central Politburo Committee printed an official document to call for the mobilization and discipline of party organs across the country in a fight against the pandemic, demanding that party members should take up the fight as 'a political mission' (The State Council of the People's Republic of China 2020). This document set in motion a flurry of articles to propagate the predominant significance of the Party's political leadership to the controlling and preventing of the pandemic, as well as campaigns, which were termed 'fast-track-dismissal', to purge and punish local cadres. During February 2020, 5 cadres were held accountable and punished each day on average. Although the number of cadres disciplined dropped significantly in March, there were as many as 3000 cadres disciplined by 15 March 2020. In Hubei province, two top senior officials—Jiang Chaoliang (Hubei's Communist Party chief) and Ma Guoqiang (Wuhan's Communist Party chief) were dismissed.

The administrative accountability system of China has been driven by, and evolved with, crises of human security. But, it would be wrong to assume that the COVID-19 pandemic has pushed the government to improve civil engagement or public accountability. Although the pandemic snapped the central government into a campaign to discipline local state cadres, the party-state-society triangle has not been altered. It is fair to say that local officials have been working tirelessly and scrupulously in support of China's human security during the pandemic. But, evaluationally, they remained accountable to their superior, rather than the citizens they served. Legally, the state apparatus retained the monopoly on the power to supervise and discipline cadres (see: Ministry of Justice of the People's Republic China 2018). The power to inspect and supervise misbehaviours of cadres during the pandemic was endowed almost exclusively, as always, to the Central Commission for Discipline Inspection (the CCDI) and the affiliated local branches. The civil society was not legally vested with any right to hold officials accountable unless via channels provided by the CCID. For instance, recent statistical research shows that 97% of the public accounting practices between 21 January and 5 March 2020 were conducted by 'party and government organs' (Bao 2020, 202).

Management of social opinions. Going hand in hand with the punishment of the local state cadres was the management of public opinion, especially on the Internet. Already in *The Regulation on the Urgent Handling of Public Health Emergencies* of 2006, the central government stated the necessity of 'psychological intervention' in public health crisis (The Central Government of the PRC 2006). The art of steering the heart and mind of the people was crucial to the CCP's legitimation during the COVID-19 pandemic, as more than 1 billion netizens in China, under the policy of social distancing, were anxiously imbibing information on screen, on not a daily but minutely basis.

Renmin Ribao, in an opinion piece, argued that the government must have a stronger response to social opinion amid the pandemic (*Renmin Ribao* 2020a). But the paradigm of the social opinion work was not about answering to the civic demand for policy changes; rather, it was about funnelling the emotional outbursts of the public mind amid a crisis. In a manner not unlike how the WHO defined the public health emergency response guide, *Renmin Ribao* mapped out a scrupulous guide for containing social opinion crises, which, depending on the severity and intensity, were grouped into four levels: the normal, the sensitive, the important, and the extremely severe (*Renmin Ribao* 2020b). In the last category—the extremely severe social opinion crisis—the government is advised to 'initiate an emergency plan and respond quickly to contain and control the risk' (ibid.).

The way the central authority handled the crisis of Li Wenliang's death is a case in point. In December 2019, Li Wenliang, a 34-year-old doctor in Wuhan, warned his colleague of COVID-19 privately on the social media app but was censored and reprimanded by the local police for 'spreading rumours'. He died of COVID-19 on 7 February 2020, causing a whirlwind of public criticisms against the censorship system and the lack of freedom of speech in China. Considering the death of Li Wenliang as a major blow to public confidence, the central authority quickly intervened to channel public sentiment. On 7 February, the CCDI established a task force to investigate Li Wenliang's death. In early March, the CCDI issued a public notice declaring that they 'ordered the local police to retract the admonishment letter', and, in the following month, punished the deputy director of the police station and the policeman for wrongly reprimanding Li Wenliang (Wuhan Police Station 2020). Meanwhile, Li Wenliang was posthumously awarded ceremonial recognitions for his sacrifice as a frontline medical worker. There are still a great number of netizens recognizing Li Wenliang as a 'whistle blower', and, by making tributes to his death, protested the state's suppression of the freedom of speech. As a result, Li Wenliang's social network account became a digital mourning site with more than one million comments. However, politically sensitive discourses were removed from his blogposts and the anti-establishment discourses built around Li Wenliang were diluted by competing narratives, including the more neutral narratives that described Li Wenliang as a young professional, and the more nationalistic narratives that criticized the anti-establishment discourses for supplying foreigners with materials to besmirch China's international image. If the local police of Wuhan, which reprimanded Li Wenliang along with 7 of his colleagues for 'spreading rumours', represented an Orwellian authoritarian state heavy-handedly clamping down on the freedom of speech with advanced technology, the central government's effort to manoeuvre social opinions was much subtler.

Draconic mobilization against the pandemic. Apart from punishing state cadres and channelling societal dissatisfaction, the central authority put in place draconic but highly effective mobilization against the pandemic. This assured that the central authority could present and claim themselves as the only reliable and robust provider of human security for the Chinese society.

The massive mobilization started with what IR scholars term 'securitization', a process 'through which an intersubjective understanding is constructed within a political community to treat something as an existential threat to a valued referent object, and to enable a call for urgent and exceptional measures to deal with the threat' (Buzan and Wæver 2003, 491). As soon as the lockdown of Wuhan was declared, the discourses around the COVID-19 in newspapers and the social media came to be a wash with security jargons: local cadres were likened as 'military personnel' who should have 'discipline' on the 'frontline' and 'battleground'; masks, disinfectants, and coveralls were metaphorized as 'ammunition' and 'supplies'; doing research on the virus was described as 'reconnoitering the enemy' (see: *Hubei Ribao* 2020). When Vice Premier Sun Chunlan visited the 'medical frontline' of Wuhan on 7 February 2020, she urged Wuhan government to control the virus and secure health security of the people as if in 'wartime state' (Hu and Zhao 2020). Four days later on 11 February, Xi Jinping, making historical references to the Maoist military strategy, described the campaign against the pandemic as 'People's War' (Ren and Wu 2020).

Following Wuhan, several northern cities, such as Beijing, Dalian, Baoding, declared their entry into 'wartime state', allowing the central- and local authority to mobilize resources and manpower to administer, without legal proceedings, swift restrictions on resident's movements, temperature checking, and nucleic acid tests, all on a massive scale. Wartime narratives were widely propagated in the rural area of Hubei province, to publicize the threat of COVID-19 to health security (He et al. 2020, 252). In the more urbanized Wuhan, some 7000 volunteers were recruited in less than 12 hours, to deliver goods, check residents' body temperature, and promote the central authority's presence at the grass-root level. The central government also tasked 19 provinces with assisting 16 prefectural cities in Hubei, at the critical time when Hubei suffered from material shortages. Privately owned mega-corporations also aligned themselves with the state's call for assisting Wuhan. Tecent and Alibaba, respectively, donated cash and materials worth 1.5 billion and 1 billion RMB (Wang et al. 2020b).

As part of the national mobilization efforts, state-owned enterprises (SOEs) were requested by the central authority to participate in disaster relief missions, with orders given in non-negotiable terms. On 30 January, the State-owned Assets Supervision and Administration Commission of the State Council (SASAC), a special commission under the State Council and responsible for managing SOEs, instructed SOEs to 'shoulder responsibilities in responding to the virus', supplying Wuhan with electricity, medical equipment, food, and particularly manpower. On 23 January, some 40,000 construction workers and staff in Wuhan were assembled by the China State Construction Engineering Corporation into building two emergency specialty field hospitals for temporary treatment of patients with COVID-19. The construction of the two makeshift hospitals was completed at a breathtaking speed within 10 days, symbolizing the mobilization efficiency of the CCP.

Human Security as the Master-Signifier in the Legitimation Process

Embedding its legitimation process in the master-signifier of human security, the CCP not only secured its legitimacy, but also deepened its reach of power into China's economic- and societal structure. The 'master-signifier' is a signifier that confers meaning to other words and discourses (Žižek 1989, 58). If democracy is the master-signifier in American politics, then human security is the master-signifier in China's campaign against the pandemic. In politics, a social actor or a social group that occupies the master-signifier is enchanted with more moral and social capital to advance its political agenda than those who do not. In the name of protecting human security, the top leadership of China was able to further the strategic agenda in economic reform as well as social governance.

Economically, the massive mobilization against the pandemic was an opportunity for the SOE reform, allowing the CCP to claim more leadership over the SOEs in the name of disaster relief. Since taking office in 2013, Xi has been eager to have the SOEs play a greater role in support of the state's strategic and social policies. The SOEs, with their laggard managerial structure, occupied around 28% of China's industrial assets but delivered only 18% of total output. From the current administration's perspective, they were neither competitive in the market nor instrumental to the public. But, if the Xi administration had to tolerate a stagnation of the SOE reform due to bureaucratic inertia during his first term, then the COVID-19 crisis offered an irrefutable ground to justify a restructuring of the production activities as well as personnel arrangements of the SOEs, pushing forward the reform agenda faster than would be.

Already in 2015, the major SOE reform policy document had ceased to mention 'the decisive role for markets in resource allocation' (The State Council of People's Republic of China 2015). The shift of the Party's centrality in economic management away from the 'invisible hand' towards the 'visible hand' has been more pronounced in 2020 and 2021. In an important speech in February 2020, Xi highlighted the importance to 'strengthen macro-control as a hedge against the impact of the pandemic' and to 'cement the party's leadership…in socio-economic development' (Xi 2020a). The path towards more socio-political involvement in the SOEs was further concretized in May 2021, when the SASAC, with increased powers to supervise Chinese SOEs, announced in an official document that 'we will improve the Party's leadership in all aspects of the SOE management' (SASAC 2021).

It was also in the name of human security that the CCP justified the implementation of the much disreputable urban grid management system (*wanggehua guanli*), a net-based surveillance system developed in 2014 to provide services to citizens as well as security for the state, mostly in the form of human surveillance. Although the urban grid management system, from the Western perspective, is a sign of police state, it arguably did contribute to the infectious disease prevention work by detecting the flow of population, a task crucial to the control of the coronavirus. During the pandemic, as many as 4.5 million social workers operated with the system day and night to locate where the residents have been and check their body temperature (Liu 2020). Augmented with advanced security protection technology, the system 'can identify where people gather and will inform social workers instantaneously to advise them apart through radio' (Yu 2020).

Although the idea and practice of population surveillance were far from being uncontroversial, concerns over violation of privacy were justified, and put aside indefinitely, on grounds of human security. Facial recognition technology, planted to halt the spread of COVID-19, has become a new normal in residential communities in China. Scanning a coloured code on the phone to prove one's health credential is now a must for visitors to public facilities. Tracking technology has never been so intrusive, effective, and ubiquitous. Augmented with the power conferred by the master-signifier of human security, the party-state was allowed to turn what used to be an egragious symbol of authoritarianism into a technical solution to the risk society. *The Global Times*, a state-run tabloid, touted, with a new-found pride, that the urban grid management system 'enables nationwide instructions, policies and rules to reach every resident'. Rather than 'an authoritarian machine designed to keep surveillance on people', it was a 'modernized governance innovation in China' that 'helps fight coronavirus' (*The Global Times* 2020).

The contrast between China and the United States in their performance of containing the pandemic was seen as the best and a lasting vindication of the CCP's legitimacy. By 22 May 2021, according to WHO, there were as many as 32,706,250 people infected with the coronavirus in the United States—a bleak number three hundred times greater than that in China. For observers from Western democracies, China's heavy-handed, whole-of-society approach to the pandemic shifted away from a material for criticisms, towards a lesson to learn from, if not a model to follow. Jürgen Gerhards and Michael Zürn, professors of the

Free University of Berlin, wrote of China becoming 'a clear winner when it comes to the mastering of the COVID-19 pandemic' (Gerhards and Zürn 2021). In terms of managing public health security and overcoming socio-economic consequences of the crisis, the West lost its claim on the performance superiority to China. While the Chinese management of the crisis could hardly discredit the legitimacy of Western democracy, the contrast between China, whose economic activities came back to normal in 2021, and the United States, whose citizens remained resistant to a collectivist response to the pandemic, offered the Chinese central government a compelling narrative to buttress popular faith and confidence in China's model of governance (Zhao 2020); hence the continuation of the CCP's legitimacy.

The New York Times, in an opinion piece in February 2020, wrote of the pandemic as a sign that 'shows China's governance failure' (Li 2020). But what happened in the following months proved that the columnist might have made too bold a claim. China's political system, characterized by the party-state-society triangle, is conducive to crises of human security, and has been a major institutional cause, between late December 2019 and early January 2020, of the mishandling of the COVID-19 in Wuhan. But paradoxically, it was also through the party-state-society triangle—whereby the central authority attributed blame to local cadres, manipulated societal opinions, and mobilized the whole society against the virus—that the CCP restored its legitimacy, boosted citizens' confidence in China's governance model, and tightened its grip on the economic and societal governance in the name of human security.

Concluding Remarks

I have demonstrated how the 'party-state-society triangle' was paradoxically both a cause of and a solution to crises of human security; how the CCP preserved its legitimacy, not despite but because of, the COVID-19 pandemic; and how the leadership of the CCP, by appropriating the master-signifier of human security, strengthened control over social governance and pushed for economic reforms. I now conclude the chapter with a dialogue with scholarships on the CCP's legitimacy.

Scholars in China study have been perplexed by the longevity of the CCP, whose dominance has endured for more than 70 years without electoral democracy. The durability of the CCP's legitimacy has challenged the three ideal types of legitimacy as defined by Marx Weber: the traditional (that people obey a regime because of their habit), the charismatic (that people obey a regime out of their affection toward the leader), and the legal/rational (that people obey a regime because doing so is beneficial to them on the basis of economic calculation or/and legal reasoning). Clearly, since the Republican era, China was broken away from its feudalist past, and the mandate of heaven a had descended into an object of historical reflection rather than a source of political authority; no leader after Mao Zedong could ever command the same charisma to mobilize the bureaucrats and the society; few would agree that the rule of law has a discernible place in Chinese politics, though the current administration has publicly espoused it. So how come that the CCP maintained its legitimacy even in the face of famine, extreme poverty, and other disasters such as the COVID-19?

The most common answer to this question is to attribute the resilience of the CCP's legitimacy to the miraculous economic performance it delivered in the reform era. Zhao Dingxin argues that Weber's formulation did not include 'performance legitimacy'—a 'pragmatic rationality' that 'shaped people's understanding of the power of the rulers and the state in Chinese political culture' (Zhao 2009, 420). It 'pushes China's top officials to work harder, behave like moral leaders of the society, and bring measurable benefits to the people' (ibid., 427). We may understand 'performance legitimacy' as 'meritocracy of the Emperor'. Further, Zhao elaborates that the heavy reliance on government performance can be dangerous for the CCP, because 'if the state becomes unable to live up to popular expectations, the government and regime will be in crisis' (ibid., 428).

Elizabeth Perry, perhaps the most renowned scholar in the field of CCP studies, disagrees with Zhao, contending that Zhao's argument wrongly confuses what is instrumental and what is morally desirable (Perry 2018). What legitimacy means, Perry argues, is that people have moral appeals to the governance of a party, even in the face of 'unfavourable performance'. A regime is legitimate when it has a moral right to rule (ibid., 15). For Perry, the CCP used to be a moral ruler, but now, she suggests, the CCP's ruling legitimacy derives mainly from rewriting the past records to cast the current regime in a favourable light, and, in Xi's era, the CCP's historical legitimacy is 'in danger of depleted by current governance practices' (ibid., 17). But apart from throwing criticisms at the CCP's deplorable practice of wrapping itself in the mantle of historical legitimacy, Perry falls short of offering any definitive answer as to why, let alone how, the CCP's ruling remains unshakable. If Zhao confuses instrumentality and morality, Perry confuses what ought to be and what is. Unable to resolve the is-and-ought problem, Perry admittedly says that 'there is…no surefire signal of an authoritarian regime's imminent loss of legitimacy; the only definitive proof lies in its demise' (ibid., 18).

I am convinced that both Zhao and Perry are misguided, and misguiding, in their enquiry into the question regarding the CCP's legitimacy, for two reasons. First, both Zhao and Perry assume legitimacy to be static, ideal, rather than a dynamic process. This problem is pointed out by Peter Sandby-Thomas, who calls for shifting our focus away from legitimacy from legitimation, replacing 'legitimacy's claims of causality and certainty by legitimation's acknowledgment of complexity and contingency' (Sandby-Thomas 2014, 585). Legitimacy-building is not static. It is a dynamic process involving contentions and activities. Analysing the CCP through a static lens, Zhao and Perry are unnecessarily preoccupied with slapping the CCP's governance practices on some a prior categories, that is, Weber's three forms of legitimacy. Their starting point is not entirely convincing. Their analysis is based on the assumption that a regime is legitimate only when its state of being conforms to some pre-established utopia. But this is not what Weber meant. When Weber formulated the three ideal types of legitimacy, he intended to create some heuristic devices to shed light on political obedience, rather than to essentialize what a legitimate regime is or to give a normative account on what it should be.

Second, Zhao and Perry overlook how the party and the state in China were separated from each other in the CCP's legitimation process. They assume that the Party and the state are unified, and, on that basis, tend to see the dichotomous and potentially antagonistic relationship between the party-state and the society. The corollary contradicted the strong popular support for the CCP despite unfavourable governance performance (Wu et al. 2021). The crucial aspect that they miss is how the party and the state are politically different entities. Whereas the state is an administrative apparatus or a bureaucratic machine vested with executive function, the political power lies with the party.

Zheng Yongnian hints that understanding the CCP requires us to see not a dualistic relationship between the party-state and the society, but a three-way dialectics between the party, the state, and the society (Zheng 2009). Zheng's theorization implies that the CCP, acting as the central government, can build up legitimacy by embodying itself as an arbitor who reconciles conflicts between the local authority and the society in the face of social crises. Philips Kuhn, in his classic book *Soul-stealers,* makes a similar point. Kuhn argues that crises fueled, rather than frustrated, the political system of imperial China (Kuhn 1990). Whereas the bureaucrats held routine power, the Emperor exercised arbitrary power, which allowed him to mobilize the bureaucrats in abnormal situations (such as the sorcery crisis), to further his authority over the bureaucrats, whose routine power was normally out of his control. When Zheng Yongnian calls the CCP the 'organization emperor' of China, he means that the CCP exercises arbitary power as a Chinese Emperor to maintain its legitimacy. Crises were as necessary for the CCP to maintain its legitimacy in the COVID-19 pandemic of 2020–2021 as they were for Qianlong Emperor to extend his patrimonial power into the bureaucrats in the Sorcery Scare of 1768.

There is, therefore, a historical continuity in the legitimation logic inherent to the political governance in China from the Qing dynasty through to the modern day. Just as how the Sorcery Scare revealed a fundamental issue in the system of bureaucratic monarchy, the COVID-19 pandemic revealed a fundamental issue in the party-state system, namely, the party-state-society triangle, a political-cultural structure that is simultaneously a cause of and the solution to system crises. Perry, in a book published in 2018, asks the Chinese. What legitimated the CCP should be examined on a case-by-case basis, attentive to the context on the ground, rather than on some pre-established ethical notion about legitimacy. In the COVID-19 pandemic, it was not the CCP's moral appeal, but its capacity to deliver, and exploit the discursive power of, human security, that saved the party-state's reputation. If the CCP's legitimation is fuelled by crises of human security, then we are looking to expect the consolidation, rather than the demise, of the lasting reign of China's organizational emperor.

References

Bachman, D., & Bachman, D. M. (2006). *Bureaucracy, economy, and leadership in China: The institutional origins of the Great Leap Forward*. Cambridge University Press.

Bao, Kun. (2020). AI-enhanced legal response to pandemic crisis 重大疫情背景下的人工智能法治应对. In: Yandong. Cui, ed., *The Blue book of world artificial intelligence rule of law* 世界人工智能法治蓝皮书. Shanghai: Association of Shanghai Legal Studies.

Buzan, B., & Wæver, O. (2003). *Regions and powers: The structure of international security*. London: Cambridge University Press.

Caixin. (2019). Wuhan reports 27 cases of viral pneumonia, the source of virus still under investigation 武汉通报27例病毒性肺炎疫情 病原检测正在进行. *Caixin* [online]. 31 December 2019. [Viewed 28 March 2021]. Available from: https://www.caixin.com/2019-12-31/101499761.html.

Caixin. (2020). Mayor of Wuhan admitted untimely information disclosure 武汉市长承认前期信息披露不及时 [online]. *Caixin*. 27 January 2019. [Viewed 28 March 2021]. https://china.caixin.com/2020-01-27/101508817.html.

Crete-Nishihata, Masashi, Dalek, Jakub, Knockel, Jeffrey, Lawford, Nicola, Wesley, Caroline, & Zhou, Mari. (2020). Censored contagion II a timeline of information control on Chinese social media during COVID-19. *The Citizen Lab* [online]. 25 August 2020. [Viewed 22 March 2021] Available from: https://citizenlab.ca/2020/08/censored-contagion-ii-a-timeline-of-information-control-on-chinese-social-media-during-covid-19/.

Chan, L. H., Chen, L., & Xu, J. (2012). China's engagement with global health diplomacy: Was SARS a watershed? In *Negotiating and navigating global health: Case studies in global health diplomacy* (pp. 203–219).

Davidson, Helen. (2020). First Covid-19 case happened in November, China government records show—report [online]. *The Guardian*. 13 March 2020. [Viewed 13 April 2021]. Available from: https://www.theguardian.com/world/2020/mar/13/first-covid-19-case-happened-in-november-china-government-records-show-report.

Fan, Wei. (2020). Medical staff of the central hospital of Wuhan tell the truth: The pandemic is a demon-revealing mirror 武汉市中心医院医护人员吐真情：疫情是面照妖镜 [online]. *Global Times*. 16 March 2020. [Viewed 29 March 2021]. Available from: https://www.medsci.cn/article/show_article.do?id=2f19190169f7.

Foucault, M. (1990). *The history of sexuality: An introduction, volume I*. Trans. Robert Hurley (p. 95). New York: Vintage.

Freedman, A. (2005). SARS and regime legitimacy in China. *Asian Affairs*, *36*(2), 169–180.

Gao, J. (2015). Pernicious manipulation of performance measures in China's cadre evaluation system. *The China Quarterly*, 618–637.

Gerhards, Jürgen, & Zürn, Michael. (2021). China gewinnt im Systemvergleich. *Frankfurter Allgemeine Zeitung* [online]. 13 January 2021. [Viewed on 10 April 2021]. Available from: https://www.faz.net/aktuell/karriere-hochsc

hule/china-gewinnt-im-systemvergleich-bei-corona-pandemie-bewaeltigung-17141504.html?GEPC=s9&premium=0xd860954a2bafb95fa35e9100ee5fde1c#void.

Global Times. (2020). Community grid system helps China fight virus [online]. *The Global Times*. 5 February 2020. [Viewed on 5 May 2021]. Available from: https://www.globaltimes.cn/content/1178528.shtml.

Hameiri, S., & Jones, L. (2016). Rising powers and state transformation: The case of China. *European Journal of International Relations*, 22(1), 72–98.

He, A. J., Shi, Y., & Liu, H. (2020). Crisis governance, Chinese style: Distinctive features of China's response to the Covid-19 pandemic. *Policy Design and Practice*, *3*(3), 242–258.

Hubei Ribao. (2020). Wartime conduct in wartime condition "战时"状态要有"战时"作为 [online]. *Hubei Ribao*. 1 February 2020. [Viewed 30 February 2020]. Available from: https://epaper.hubeidaily.net/pc/content/202002/01/content_20139.html.

Human Security Unit. (2013). *Lessons from the field: Applying the human security approach through the United Nations trust fund for human security*. New York: United Nations Trust Fund for Human Security & Human Security Unit OCHA.

Hu, Hao, & Zhao, Wenjun. (2020). Instruction team from the central government to Wuhan: Control the pandemic in wartime state 中央赴湖北指导组: 以战时状态全力抓好源头防控 [online]. *The State Council of People's Republic of China*. 7 February 2020. [Viewed 28 March 2021]. Available from: http://www.gov.cn/guowuyuan/2020-02/06/content_5475425.htm.

Kuhn, P. A. (1990). *Soulstealers: The Chinese sorcery scare of 1768*. Cambridge, MA: Harvard University Press.

Li, Yuan. (2020). Coronavirus crisis shows China's governance failure [online]. *The New York Times*. 4 February 2020. [Viewed 28 April 2021]. Available from: https://www.nytimes.com/2020/02/04/business/china-coronavirus-government.html.

Li, W., & Yang, D. T. (2005). The great leap forward: Anatomy of a central planning disaster. *Journal of Political Economy*, *113*(4), 840–877.

Liao, Jun, & Le, Wenwan. (2020). The epidemic preventable and controllable—Answers to questions about the prevention and control of the Novel Coronavirus in Wuhan 疫情可防可控——武汉市就新型冠状病毒感染的肺炎综合防控工作答记者问 [online]. *Xinhuashe*. 19 January 2020. [Viewed 29 March 2021]. Available from: https://baijiahao.baidu.com/s?id=1656131702921143315&wfr=spider&for=pc.

Liao, Jun, & Li, Changzheng. (2020). Expert says the pneumonia of unknown etiology in Wuhan is preventable and controllable 专家称武汉不明原因的病毒性肺炎可防可控 [online]. *Xinhuashe*. 11 January 2020. [Viewed on 13 April 2020]. Available from: https://www.chinanews.com/sh/2020/01-11/9056969.shtml.

Liu, Ziyang. (2020). 4.5 million grid management workers at the frontline of campaign against the pandemic 450万网格员筑牢疫情社区防控"第一道防线" [online]. *Legal Daily*. 10 March 2020. [Viewed 29 March 2021]. Available from: http://www.legaldaily.com.cn/index/content/2020-03/10/content_8138243.htm.

Ministry of Justice of the People's Republic China. (2018). *Supervision law of the People's Republic of China* 中华人民共和国监察法 [online]. Ministry of Justice of the People's Republic China. 25 December 2018 [Viewed on 2 May 2020]. Available from: http://www.moj.gov.cn/Department/content/2018-12/25/357_182295.html.

NHC. (2007). National plan for case surveillance, investigation and management of Pneumonia of unknown Etiology (PUE) 中华人民共和国国家卫生和计划生育委员会. 全国不明原因肺炎病例监测、排查和管理方案 [online]. *National Health and Family Planning Commission of PRC*. 6 August 2007. [Viewed on 15 April 2020]. Available from: http://www.nhc.gov.cn/bgt/pw10708/200708/4455f46a2f5e4908a8561c079ecbcf0e.shtml.

Perry, Elizabeth. (2018). Is the Chinese communist regime legitimate? *The China Questions: Critical Insights into a Rising Power*, ed. Jennifer Rudolph Michael Szonyi, 11–17.

Renmin Ribao. (2020a). Zhongnanshan: Novel Coronavirus human-to-human transmissible, SARS crisis not to be repeated 钟南山: 新型肺炎存在人传人现象, 不会重复SARS疫情 [online]. *Renmin Ribao*. 20 January 2020. [Viewed on 15 April 2020]. Available from: https://baijiahao.baidu.com/s?id=1656327014730039963&wfr=spider&for=pc.

Renmin Ribao. (2020b). The level of response to the pandemic has been lowered, but we cannot downscale the management of social opinion 疫情应急响应等级下调 舆情风险管理不能下调 [online]. *Renmin Ribao*. 10 March 2020. [Viewed on 15 April 2020]. Available from: http://yuqing.people.com.cn/n1/2020/0310/c209043-31625854.html.

Ren, Yilin, & Wu, Zhaofei. (2020). Xi Jinping: Constructing the people's defense line a key to the war against the pandemic. 决胜战"疫"重中之重 习近平强调构筑疫情防控的人民防线 [online]. *CCP News*. 11 February 2020. Available from: http://theory.people.com.cn/n1/2020/0211/c40531-31580687.html.

Rogaski, R. (2004). *Hygienic modernity*. University of California Press.

Sandby-Thomas, P. (2014). How do you solve a problem like legitimacy? Contributing to a new research agenda. *Journal of Contemporary China*, *23*(88), 575–592.

SASAC. (2021). SASAC enterprise reform Bureau Action Plan of 2021. 国资委企业改革局2021年工作安排 [online]. *SASAC*. 23 March 2021. [Viewed on 8 March 2021]. Available from: http://www.sasac.gov.cn/n2588030/n2588924/c17725438/content.html.

The Central Government of the PRC. (2006). Regulation on the urgent handling of public health emergencies 国家突发公共卫生事件应急预案 [online]. *The Central Government of the People's Republic of China*. 26 February 2006. [Viewed on 28 April]. Available from: http://www.gov.cn/yjgl/2006-02/26/content_211654.htm.

The Paper. (2020). In-depth report: How the web-based reporting system failed on the even of the pandemic 深度 | 疫情初期, 网络直报系统在武汉为何失灵了? [online]. 15 March 2020. [Viewed 24 October 2020]. Available from: https://www.thepaper.cn/newsDetail_forward_6523974.

The State Council Information Office of the People's Republic of China. (2020). *Fighting Covid-19 China in action*. Beijing: Foreign Languages Press.

The State Council of the People's Republic of China. (2015). China issues guideline to deepen SOE reforms [online]. *Xinhuashe* [Viewed 23 December 2020]. Available from: http://english.www.gov.cn/policies/latest_releases/2015/09/13/content_281475189210840.htm.

The State Council of the People's Republic of China. (2020). The notice on strengthening the party's leadership and providing political reassurances to win the battle of infectious disease containment《关于加强党的领导、为打赢疫情防控阻击战提供坚强政治保证的通知》. [online]. *Xinhuashe* [Viewed 22 December 2020]. Available from: http://www.gov.cn/zhengce/2020-01/28/content_5472753.htm.

Thornton, P. M. (2009). Crisis and governance: SARS and the resilience of the Chinese body politic. *The China Journal*, (61), 23–48.

Tian, Qiaoping, & Chen, Zhuo. (2020). Zhang Jixian, the first doctor to make the right judgment about and report to the authority the pandemic: I shed tears of my entire life 最早判断出疫情并上报的医生张继先: 这次把一生的泪流光了. *Changjiang Ribao* [online]. 7 February 2020. [Viewed on 15 April 2020]. Available from: https://www.ccdi.gov.cn/lswh/renwu/202002/t20200207_210984.html.

Wang, L., Wang, Y., Yang, G., Ma, J., Wang, L., & Qi, X. (2013). China information system for disease control and prevention (CISDCP). *HIT Briefing Book*, 101–108.

Wang, Yu, Xing, Nijuan, Ni, Daxin, Li, Qun., & Feng, Zijian. (2017). Performance of surveillance system of pneumonia with unknown etiology in two hospitals at municipal (prefecture) level in Anhui province. *Disease Surveillance* 疾病监测, *32*(5), 428–432.

Wang, Pin, Lu, Bo, Sun, Fei, Zhao, Bo, & Zheng, Wenbin. (2020a). Care for national health for the future of medical work: Speeches of guests attending Boao Global Health Forum on the welfare of human health关注全民健康打造未来医疗 ————出席博鳌亚洲论坛全球健康论坛大会的嘉宾共话人类健康福祉 [online]. 14 June 2019. Qingdao Ribao [cited in China CDC, viewed 1 May 2021]. Available from: http://www.chinacdc.cn/mtbd_8067/201906/t20190614_203242.html.

Wang, Xiaona, Shen, Haiyan, Jia, Lu, Zou, Wenrong. (2020b). Report on corporate donations to China's anti-Coronavirus campaign 中国抗击新冠肺炎疫情企业捐赠报告 [online]. *Jiemian*. 10 March 2020. [Viewed 23 March 2021]. Available from: https://www.jiemian.com/article/4086815.html.

Wemheuer, F. (2010). Dealing with responsibility for the great leap famine in the People's Republic of China. *China Quarterly*, 176–194.

Wishnick, E. (2010). Dilemmas of securitization and health risk management in the People's Republic of China: The cases of SARS and avian influenza. *Health Policy and Planning*, *25*(6), 454–466.

Whiting, S. H. (2017). The cadre evaluation system at the grass roots: The paradox of party rule. In *Critical readings on the Communist Party of China (4 Vols. Set)* (pp. 461–478). Brill.

Wuhan Government. (2019). Wuhan police: Do not spread rumours! Eight rumourmonger dealt with by police in conformity to legal provision 武汉公安机关: 莫传谣!8名散布谣言者被警方依法查处 [online]. *Wuhan Government*. 1 January 2020. [Viewed 15 May 2021]. Available from: https://www.hubei.gov.cn/zxjy/rdhy/202001/t20200101_1862068.shtml.

Wuhan Police Station. (2020). Wuhan police station to punish staff responsible for reprimanding Li Wenliang武汉市公安局对李文亮医生被训诫一案相关责任人作出处理. http://www.xinhuanet.com/politics/2020-03/19/c_1125737967.htm.

Wu, C., Shi, Z., Wilkes, R., Wu, J., Gong, Z., He, N., & Nicola Giordano, G. (2021). Chinese citizen satisfaction with government performance during COVID-19. *Journal of Contemporary China*, 1–15.

WMHC. (2019). WMHC bulletin on the Pneumonia with unknown Etiology in our city 武汉市卫健委关于当前我市肺炎疫情的情况通报 [online]. *Wuhan Municipal Health Commission*. 31 December 2019. [Viewed 28 February 2021]. Available from: http://wjw.wuhan.gov.cn/gsgg/202004/t20200430_1199576.shtml.

WMHC. (2020a). WMHC bulletin on the Pneumonia with unknown Etiology 武汉市卫生健康委员会关于不明原因的病毒性肺炎情况通报 [online]. 5 January 2020. *Wuhan Municipal Health Commission*. [Viewed 28 February 2021]. Available from: http://wjw.wuhan.gov.cn/gsgg/202004/t20200430_1199589.shtml

WMHC. (2020b). Q&A on the Novel Coronavirus (14 January 2020) 新型冠状病毒感染的肺炎疫情知识问答 (2020年1月14日) [online]. *Wuhan Municipal Health Commission*. 14 January 2020. [Viewed 28 February 2021]. Available from: http://wjw.wuhan.gov.cn/gsgg/202004/t20200430_1199594.shtml.

Xi, Jinping. (2020a). Xi Jinping: Speech on the conference about the deployment to push for Coronavirus control and prevention and socio-economic development 习近平: 在统筹推进新冠肺炎疫情防控和经济社会发展工作部署会议上的讲话 [online]. *Xinhuashe*. 23 February 2020. [Viewed 6 April 2021]. Available at: http://www.gov.cn/xinwen/2020-02/24/content_5482502.htm.

Xi, Jinping. (2020b). Speech at the Central Politburo standing committee conference on measures to address the Novel Coronavirus 在中央政治局常委会会议研究应对新型冠状病毒肺炎疫情工作时的讲话 [online]. *Qiushi*. 3 January 2020. [Viewed 24 October 2020]. Available from: http://www.qstheory.cn/dukan/qs/2020-02/15/c_1125572832.htm.

Xinhuanet, (2020). How the alarm was raised—Zhang Jixian, the first to report the epidemic 警报是这样拉响的——对话"疫情上报第一人"张继先 [online]. *Liaowang*. 20 April 2020. [Viewed 25 March 2021]. Available from: http://www.xinhuanet.com/politics/2020-04/20/c_1125878293.htm.

Yu, Jianhui. (2020). Security protection technology in the COVID-19 pandemic. *China Security Protection Technology and Application*, *2020*(1), 20–23.

Zhang, L., Chen, K., & Zhao, J. (2020). Evidence-based decision-making for a public health emergency in China: Easier said than done. *The American Review of Public Administration*, *50*(6-7), 720–724.

Zhao, D. (2009). The mandate of heaven and performance legitimation in historical and contemporary China. *American Behavioral Scientist*, 53(3), 416–433.

Zhao, Jinzhao. (2019). Pneumonia of unknown origin found in Wuhan, local seafood market sanitized 武汉发现不明原因肺炎 当地一海鲜市场消毒 (更新). [online]. *Caixin*. 31 December 2019. [Viewed 28 March 2021]. Available from: https://www.caixin.com/2019-12-31/101499720.html.

Zhao, Xiaoyu. (2020). A discourse analysis of Quotidian expressions of nationalism during the COVID-19 pandemic in Chinese cyberspace. *Journal of Chinese political science*, 1–17.

Zheng, Yongnian. (2009). *The Chinese Communist Party as organizational emperor: Culture, reproduction, and transformation*. Routledge.

Zhou, Xueguang. (2012). Yundong xing zhili jizhi: Zhongguo guojia zhili luoji de zai sikao [The Mechanism of Campaign-style governance: Rethinking the Logic of Chinese State Governance]. *Kaifangshidai, 2012*(9), 105–125.

Zhou, Xueguang. (2020). Organizational response to COVID-19 crisis: Reflections on the Chinese bureaucracy and its resilience. *Management and Organization Review, 16*(3), July 2020, 473–484.

Žižek, S. (1989). *The sublime object of ideology*. Verso.

CHAPTER 4

Securitizing New Energy Amidst the Global Pandemic: The Chinese State and the Politics of Climate Change

Geoffrey C. Chen

Introduction

The sudden onset of COVID-19 brought about a dramatic disruption to human security, which has also unexpectedly shaped changes in the energy transition process in that the Chinese state has claimed commitment to combating global warming. The spread and (un)inhibition of the virus has to some extent caused scholars to reconsider the anthropocentric nature and concomitant changing role of the state. The academic discussion of anthropocentrism has incorporated the thinking of earth justice into the study of eco-politics. A long-ignored doctrine focusing on fragile natural subjects is gradually attracting more and more research as the virus erodes the global economy and society—the reflection on human security in the context of the sudden increase in the uncertainty

G. C. Chen (✉)
Department of China Studies, School of Humanities and Social Sciences,
Xi'an Jiaotong-Liverpool University, Suzhou, China
e-mail: chun-fung.chen@xjtlu.edu.cn

C. Zhang (ed.), *Human Security in China*,
https://doi.org/10.1007/978-981-16-4675-1_4

of the ecological system, namely on how to adjust the role of the state and its position, appearance, and adaptation in the era of ecological precarity (Foster 2013; Nyman 2018). This issue is embedded in the context of long-term climate change politics to strengthen the green security process of China's economic development. Green security is an extended discussion that is regarded as human security. To a certain extent, it provides a new discussion forum for the debates of security studies. Proponents of green security invite theorists to rethink the dual proposition of state security and human security in the global natural space. In the category of non-traditional security, researchers suggest an approach that embraces more non-state actors in process of reshaping the global community. This approach, within the paradigm of human security, provides a reflective account of security threats encountered by the potential effect of global warming. Even after years of diplomatic mediation, the repercussions of human-generated greenhouse gas emissions seem only to be getting worse. The average increase between 2000 and 2010 was 2.2%/year, even greater than the 1.3%/year between 1970 and 2000 (Dannreuther 2017, 157). The increasing destruction of the earth system by human activities has already made the global climate change regime a redundant, unsuitable system, and the rising insecurity has plagued the original business as usual of the economic structure. With the political momentum necessary for this energy transition, China has gradually become a key case due to its ambiguous role in recent years.

This phenomenon is related to China's expansion of new and alternative energies: starting in 2005, the central government started vigorously developing the regulatory rhythm of new energy. Through coordination with local governments, policy guidance, investment stimulus, and active participation of economic actors, China opened up a kind of response that seems to be rare, in three special industrial fields, namely three types of energy use and large-scale investment in non-hydro renewable energy, nuclear power, and electric vehicles. Among the renewable energy sources, wind power and photovoltaic power generation, as the frontier key industries, have shown rapid leaps in the past decade.

From 2010 to 2018, China's installed wind power capacity increased from 30.17 million kW to 18.26 million kW, while the installed solar power capacity has grown rapidly from the negligible 260 thousand kW in 2010 to 174.63 million kW, almost catching up with wind power in China. The two types of electricity together accounted for 18.9% of China's total installed power capacity at the end of 2018 (China Southern

Power Grid 2019, 5). Different from pioneering developments of renewable energy in Europe and the United States, this expansion is based on a complementary and non-competitive development process among state-owned enterprise groups and monopoly ecosystems. With such help, China has implemented installed capacity on a large scale. The installed capacity of nuclear power connected to the grid increased from 66.1 billion kilowatt-hours in 2009 to 326.9 billion kilowatt-hours in 2019 (Statista 2020). Furthermore, China's capacity for the production and diffusion of hydrogen and fuel-cell technologies is also catching up to, and may surpass, the rest of the world's market share. Chinese manufacturers supply more than 60% of such equipment. The central and local governments' investment policy objectives are based on the co-evolution of industrial policies using phased adjustments. The process by which the government guides manufacturing to maximize the creation of new industries in ecologically oriented markets was inherited from other green technology, techno-industrial governance, and economic institutional patterns that have emerged rapidly in recent years, though behind this backdrop, there is a state-centred assumption of human security. Such rhetoric of security placing "development" as the main subject of securitization issue, even though the environment and an alternative development concept have been discussed for modifying the current policy paradigm of the national economy. This means that environmental ethics and economic development must never form two opposing views in practice and rhetoric. In the context of China, the state is the primary (if not the only) moral undertaker to solve the green security threat. From this context, we can identify that the branch-level bureaucracy occupies an exclusive and active position as the energy transition process that promotes this practicality. The policy of adding new energy to its energy mix can be said to be a major strategy adopted by the Chinese government elites in the past 10 years to establish different conceived imperatives in energy security and environment protection, although that does not necessarily lead to a successful energy transition. As mentioned above, on the one hand, China is rapidly and massively expanding its renewable energy production capacity. However, on the other hand, given the economic development and limitations of traditional energy security thinking (Chen and Chen 2019), the central government's policy elites do not seem determined to revise the current economic structure radically. Policymakers have been slowly reducing China's traditional heavy dependence on petrochemical energy and incrementally implementing its energy diversification strategy. Although renewable energy sources have increased, the main consumption structure is still the same as that of other major industrial states. As with Canada, India, Australia, Russia, and other countries, fossil fuel is still the most important source of China's energy consumption.

As of the end of 2019, China's coal, oil, natural gas, and non-fossil energy sources accounted for 58, 19, 8, and 15% of total energy consumption in China, respectively (GEIDCO 2020, 4). However, what is different from the above-mentioned countries is that China, as an environmentally lagging country that has been criticized by advanced Western economies, has played the leading role in the discussion and negotiation of international environmental politics in recent years. In the recent academic literature, a new debate on environmental authoritarianism specific to ambiguous contributors to global warming has formed, especially after the United States unilaterally withdrew from the forum of global environmental governance (Mathews and Tan 2015; Chen and Lees 2019).

China's new energy sources, as the main area of contribution in the fight against global warming, has become the main supporting narrative for the Chinese national government's elites to protect the field of human security. From Hu Jingtao to Xi Jinping, the focus on global environmental politics (and differently from previous Chinese leaders) has continuously incorporated green investment projects into major international collaborative grand strategies and joint actions, and China's willingness to participate in multilateral climate governance inadvertently seems to have launched the country into an unexpected leadership role in global environmental governance (Chen and Lees 2021). In the process of continuously redefining the concept of security (Chapter 1), adherence to the path of developmental security seems to give ways to a strong central government to forge the necessary prerequisites for human security assurance, an unshakable, continuous, and customized foundations of legality often form the rhetorical promise for continuing to the state-building.

However, this new role does not seem to be able to conceal the slow progress in providing green security in domestic contexts. The lagging performance in many environmental areas such as water resources, soil pollution, air deterioration, carbon emissions, etc. does not seem to be improved by the diplomatic slogan politics of the central government for the short term or at all (Shapiro 2012). It seems that under the overall view of developmental security, risks related to personal environmental health were ignored in the competition for GDP growth. Energy, as a point of divergence that highly involves the intersection of economic, social, and political values, is the core policy area associated with a series of ambiguous collective security ideas and is often between multiple political value choices.

At least in the process of China's hydroelectric power generation, we have seen the human security situation regress under the power of government elites (McNally et al. 2009). Regarding nuclear power, as another area that is critical to the security of local residents, China seems to be unable to simply apply the definition of new energy to eliminate the risks and safety concerns under the new narrative and packaging of global warming, especially after the Fukushima accident. The industry's investment in the global nuclear power delay wave has decreased (Toke et al. 2021). As a rising country in the development of nuclear power, China has expanded its investment and expansion on a large scale in the past 10 years, and even inland nuclear power has prompted a huge discussion, which has caused many domestic and foreign observers who dream of China's nuclear power renaissance to put hope in this remote developing state. However, unexpectedly, many political risks caused the government elites to decrease the expansion rate.

In addition, it seems that few commentators and policymakers have pointed out the difference in social and technical perceptions between the three main energy sources under the so-called "new" energy semantics, let alone in the ambiguous "Chinese-style" human security discourses: to what extent does alternative energy as the political frontier of climate change form an institutional evolution along with the changes of context? In this chapter, I will compare and contrast the development of climate technology policies and the outcomes of industrial evolution of three new energy sectors through the analytical framework of human and green security, as well as unfold such governments' and enterprises' actions and relations in the trajectory of sectoral development. An overarching research question in this chapter is how we can identify the institutional continuity and changes of three strategic emerging sectors (renewable energy, nuclear energy, and green vehicles) within the context of COVID-19.

Renewable Energy: Wind and Solar

Wind and solar power, as the most successful non-hydropower renewable resources in recent years, has become a major new measure to address the urgent need of sustaining green security recognized by China and the world (REN21 2019). Since the passage of the Renewable Energy Law in 2006, China's newly installed wind power capacity has shown exponential growth. The central government has carried out resource coordination through the National Development and Reform Commission (NDRC), and the research and design cover the implementation of four different electricity prices across the country (Chen and Lees 2019). In the process of market development for solar and wind energy, the first policy idea was regarding how to reduce the then high equipment costs through economies of scale. The cultivation of wind and solar equipment manufacturers started from 2006, starting from a non-Western environmental governance orthodoxy policy paradigm, that is, a top-down institutional change. They learned from trial and error that only through cultivation of the independent R&D ability of local manufacturers could they achieve their goals in a large-scale economy. To some extent, it seems to cater to a local economic elite's demand for grafting and Sinicizing Western discourse into its national human security model. The policy objective is thus to reduce the cost of equipment so that all people can share cheap and clean energy to meet the urgent demand for energy security. In the past 15 years, China has shown a tendency to flourish in response to policy incentives through the participation of both central and local governments and economic actors, although to some extent, this process and development approach are mostly state-centric (Nyman and Zeng 2016).

Wind power is the first successful sector among these emerging industries. The central government first carried out large-scale bidding activities in the north and northeast regions with abundant wind resources, inviting domestic investors to participate in the development. After a few years, specific protection measures were deployed through local content requirements of production—restricting foreign participants by encouraging international firms to cooperate with domestic suppliers to participate in government programmes. This series of policy initiatives marked the first take-off of the industry, and a group of new local companies with an understanding of technological innovation, such as Xinjiang Goldwind, gradually emerged in the international market (Yip and McKern 2016).

Similar policy support then appeared in the planning of solar power generation. We have seen similar policies and measures to boost wind power generation, such as the feed-in tariff policies adopted from European countries and subsidies, as well as integrating various institutional incentives and local actors' behaviours (Chen and Lees 2019).

One of the core issues related to energy studies in China is awareness about administrative decentralization. The debate on decentralization not only involves the core basic assumptions in environmental governance, such as the need for participation and the normative foundation of market mechanisms for environmental protection, but also touches upon China's central-local relationship embedded in the institutionalization of the energy security system empirically (Nyman 2018). In the past 15 years, Chinese policy elites have placed renewable energy as a political issue at the top of the agenda. Nevertheless, it would be implausible for scholars not to talk about the model of policy decisions that have been qualitatively determined since the 1980s on China's policymaking module. The multiple, slow, and difficult-to-achieve consensus-based decision-making structures seem to define most of China's policymaking arenas, even for emerging sectors such as new energy. Indeed, in view of the outstanding performance in this field in the past 15 years, some scholars believe that fragmented authoritarianism continues to form inhibitory restrictions on the sustainable development of renewable energy and effective governance (Marks 2010). According to their view, the problem of departmentalism not only slows down the development of renewable deployment but has led to the counterattack of conventional utilities such as petrochemical energy sources (Qi et al. 2019; Ding et al. 2016), which, at the same time, has led to the challenge of inconsistent power consumption and abandonment. This policy paradigm has been reflected in the emerging field of technological innovation. However, some researchers have also emphasized that the decentralized policy experiment helps to coordinate the relationship between the central and local governments to some extent (Nahm 2017). This allows the local government to serve as a node conducive to climate technology innovation in policy formulation and policy implementation, to closing the loopholes in policy coordination in the state-led development of renewable energy (Hochstetler and Kostka 2015; Zhu et al. 2019). The centralization–decentralization argument is deeply rooted in an attempt to unearth an emerging problem in a paradox that plagues a broader sense of human security, which is related to the effort of stabilizing climate crises. How can, or should, the state play a changing role in such a trans-boundary earth system, when energy and environmental security have risen to a cross-border crisis?

An important historical moment of analysis is the green stimulus plan that the central government launched while addressing environmental (in)security after the global financial turmoil in 2008. The 12th and 13th five-year guidance documents are the first two central government policy documents to seriously promote the idea of environmental protection as a key political decision (Mathews and Tan 2015; Chen and Lees 2018). A series of policy measures were proposed during that 10-year period. This makes the renewable energy industry one of the key strategic centres for the state's deliberate cultivation, including encouraging the entry of local equipment manufacturers into the international market, the generation and consumption of renewable energy, and the export-driven green economy with drastic growth from scratch.

Many researchers are analysing the success of this field, if any, by focusing on the analysis of state intervention, including the process of policy experiments, government preferential subsidies, policy learning from successful front-running European states, trade protection measures, cooperation between local governments and entrepreneurs, the presence of state-owned enterprises, and the design of the bidding concession by the central state in the scale-up process (Lewis 2007; Gosens and Lu 2014; Toke 2017; Mathews and Tan 2014), which have been promoted internally through protectionism to form a policy market, as well as through the most important price control from the NDRC in a manner of a seemingly developmental state that introduced a series of institutionalizations of techno-governance regimes. The integration of wind and solar power generation, as Kirkegaard pointed out, forms a highly contested context. Power generators, local governments, old utilities, financiers, and domestic equipment manufacturers are embedded in a loose network involving constant negotiation among each other. In the process of public policy shaping, a state-owned enterprise-led development model with Chinese characteristics can be identified (Kirkegaard 2019, 283). Relationship politics (*guanxi*) play a subtle role in the development of renewable energy in state-sponsored sectors (Chen and Lees 2019). These discussions seem to buttress the rhetorical basis for the success of the Chinese state's global green energy growth. Although an ongoing issue is the lag of grid connection, the phenomenon of wind curtailment led to a huge waste of generated wind and solar power. Places with abundant power resources are often on the borders of China, far away from urban areas with high power demand. Some research has pointed out that the fragmented authoritarian policy model limits the central government's ability to modify this issue, which has cast a shadow over the euphoric and positive image of China as a global environmentalist (Andrews-Speed 2020; Zhang et al. 2018). For a long time, as a developing country, China's policy measures in prompting energy security have aroused criticism from many industrial economies. These protective measures related to green practices broke out during the COVID-19 epidemic and once again became criticized by many observers. First, there is the problem of lagging green power integration into the grids. Early on in the 2019 epidemic, subsidies for solar manufacturing were greatly reduced, and they were forced to compete with thermal power and other traditional petrochemical power without preparation (Gosens and Jotzo 2020). Scholars also criticized that the central government's economic stimulus measures in the post-epidemic era have not entirely focused on the green economy as stated. On the contrary, the business-as-usual is considered critical to the *sustainability of the Anthropocene* (Blühdorn 2020). The practice of such has become the political priority of the national elites. In this context, The NDRC has even cancelled subsidies for new wind power projects after 2021. The policy measures in this post-epidemic era seem to be unsatisfactory (Chen and Lees 2019; Economy 2018; Gao 2020).

In addition, some commentators have pointed out that following the COVID-19 outbreak, the Chinese government has continuously emphasized the necessity of its New Green Deal in political rhetoric, but it is still absent from policy implementation. It seems that there is not much investment so far, and much intervention is to increase the use of fossil fuels (Gosens and Jotzo 2020). Unexpectedly, the supply of solar photovoltaic subsidies has been cut off sharply since 2019. Following the COVID-19 epidemic, some of the new subsidies turned out to be part of the traditional fossil fuel energy industry. The economic setback caused by COVID-19 and the subsequent lifting measures that the country has taken for this epidemic actually seem to stand in a way similar to the narrow attitude of many contemporary development researchers proposed by Pelenc and Dubois (2020), which represents the limited view of human security, contemplating environmental issues by putting the "development" perspective on intrageneration justice rather than intergeneration justice.

In other words, the core issue of whose security we are talking about became a highly contested issue: regarding the specificity of human security and the relevant policy concerns, which security of generation deserves to be considered? Also, is that kind of security only is only related to the economic insecurity of individuals? With ambiguous definition, the boundary between human security and national security is still blurred. Scholars who support human security seem to be unable to put forward a theory that can address the above possible contradictions (Hudson et al. 2013, 28–30). Furthermore, its values related to security practices and processes have also failed to give practical meaning to the voices of actors who have not yet been represented (Nyman 2016). Although human security has lost its meaning in the evolution of the discourses and rhetoric that originated from advanced economies. It seems that it is precisely this limited concept of human security that led to a policy shift of China's new energy to solve the global energy transition crisis (Nyman 2018). Such a dilemma reflects the limited perspective in development following the COVID-19 situation. After discussing the success and failure experiences of renewable energy and its development amidst the COVID-19 outbreak for combatting global warming, we further discuss another case—nuclear power and the global energy transition imperative—to gain a more comprehensive understanding of the current institutional restructuring carried out by Chinese government elites and the institutional changes amidst the global pandemic.

Nuclear Power

Regarding alternative energy sources, the *choice* of efforts to solve climate change is actually the first to appear on the political agenda of the central government with the 10th Five-Year Guidelines. The industrial production process of nuclear power investment in the central component countries actually predates the development of policies in areas such as solar and wind energy. The development process of this policy field seems to be more dependent on the traditional centralized science and technology policy. The development logic behind it comes from a traditional energy security strategy of technological power and an international breakthrough, that is, economic nationalism.

Despite the early investment, apart from sporadic scientific and technological achievements, the scale of commercialization of nuclear power reactor technology is not substantial enough. The so-called indigenous innovation seldom has the scientific and technological output in the true sense when the slogans are introduced. Domestic reactors' research and development design is controlled by a few monopoly central state-owned enterprises led by the State-owned Assets Supervision and Administration Commission of the State Council (SASAC). However, in recent years, the Development and Reform Commission of the central government has integrated relatively dispersed resources such as nuclear power research and development and construction, while strategically inviting different advanced economies' firms to operate joint venture projects and develop new commercial nuclear power technology. A significant phenomenon that can be identified in recent developments is the emphasis on the pursuit of the latest reactors designed overseas. The industry highly relies on internationally well-known companies to conduct joint ventures in China. Most of the joint ventures involve central state-owned enterprises, and their high profile is for economic imperatives. The technology has been monopolized by two companies, namely China General Nuclear Power and China National Nuclear Corporation (CNNC).

Moreover, the policy elites have begun to consider expanding investment in the nuclear fuel cycle hierarchically. Many international cooperation projects led by central state-owned enterprises have been launched. In the past 10 years, the central state-owned enterprises have strategically invested in developing countries including Namibia, Zimbabwe, Kazakhstan, and Mongolia. They establish subsidiaries, carrying out mergers and acquisitions of overseas uranium mines and other initiatives to secure a long-term supply of resources to meet the state's imperative of self-sufficiency in its energy supply because, as some, believe uranium resources are the basis of any nuclear energy development (Zhang 2015, 61–62). Securing access to overseas uranium mines allows China to take the initiative in completing the nuclear fuel cycle. In the eleventh 5-year guideline, the State Council encouraged overseas trading of uranium from Canada, Australia, Africa, and Central Asia; central state-owned enterprises such as China National Nuclear Corporation and China General Nuclear Power Group have taken the lead in mining activities overseas (Zhou 2011, 4364). In China, satellite imaging in Lanzhou, Emeishan, and Hanzhong also shows the expansion of the nuclear industry supply base (Strategic Comments 2016). These expansions also entail the purchase of technology for reprocessing nuclear fuel from abroad to acquire the knowledge and equipment for the treatment of spent fuel at the end point of the nuclear fuel cycle. The perceived importance of investment in these devices and expertise is to increase the ability to reuse spent nuclear fuel and dispose of nuclear waste due to the deployment of new reactors.

Regarding the vexing issue of managing spent nuclear fuel produced by reactors, still no concrete and long-term solution has been offered that fits the difficult social-economic circumstance in China, although it should have been considered early on. So far, nuclear waste has not been put forward as an issue by countries around the world. Most nuclear waste is stored directly near nuclear power plant sites (Forrest and Braun 2017). In theory, as Zhou indicated, one could effectively use three approaches to manage spent fuel. Apart from the above-mentioned reprocessing and direct disposal,[1] it is suggested that one could also export spent fuel elsewhere (Zhou 2011, 4361). Most countries use direct disposal or export spent fuel to manage nuclear waste, and only about six countries have introduced reprocessing policies. China has designed a place for spent fuel storage when planning nuclear power development. However, the nuclear waste stored around the Qinshan plant, which was the first grid-connected nuclear plant in China in 1991, has surpassed the storage capacity that was foreseen when it was originally designed. Therefore, the new plan is to build a larger repository site so that storage capacity can be extended until 2025 (Zhou 2011, 4361).

However, in 2011, after the Fukushima nuclear accident, the construction of the nuclear cycle showed new twists and turns. In view of the new situation, the central government has tended to follow the trends of advanced economies, and it has begun to increase the cost of nuclear power construction for safety reasons. Such an initiative is also proposed against the backdrop of rising public awareness of the risks of nuclear power. After the incident, the public collectively asked relevant government authorities to issue more information about the development of nuclear power, and they requested more transparency in official decision-making processes (Thomson 2011). Not only did the State Council request that all nuclear power construction be suspended, but the central government-coordinated National Security Bureau, the National Energy Administration, and the China Earthquake Administration jointly invited members of the expert group of the Central Academy of Sciences to

[1] This means that the technocrats expect that the problem of nuclear waste can be solved by further extracting uranium or plutonium from the used spent energy, which requires new technology to limit the high radiation produced during the process.

conduct safety inspections for each nuclear power plant. Additionally, each nuclear power plant was required to issue short-, medium-, and long-term plans after inspection to prevent nuclear accidents like Fukushima.

It is worth noting that the long history of nuclear power development in China can be said to be contrary to the other two aforementioned development paths in new energy. Researchers have pointed out that the development of solar and wind power from scratch comes from a new kind of industrial policy, which has strengthened the functions of the central government, the authority of the central government, and the regulatory authority to some extent in line with the integration of the institutional measures of the developing state (Nahm and Steinfeld 2014; Chen and Lees 2016; Mathews and Tan 2015). Development of the industry may appear to be disorderly at the beginning. However, following a steady intervention of the central and provincial governments, a series of regulated subsidy measures for electricity prices across the country have been introduced through the promulgation of the Renewable Energy Law and a series of subsequent measures. Such regulatory interventions allow local governments to follow the policies of the leading economies to introduce supplementary subsidies and seek the adjustment of local conditions, which tend to follow or fit with the differences in local energy structure, consumption and supply, and the local contexts. In this process, the study, formulation, and implementation of policies rely on close communication with a few economic actors to facilitate the introduction of alternative energy options that achieve the energy transition in the shortest time. However, the success of alternative energy is also due to the fact that the proposed new energy has not created concerns about the interests of local or conventional utilities. The government therefore has ample room for manipulating policy choices favouring renewable energy. Compared with other so-called new energy, this hot-potato policy, in fact, depending on the context of its development, seems to be burdened by the limitations of the traditional policy model, that is, the fragmented authoritarian policy model, from its inception to the present day (Toke et al. 2021). On the one hand, civil nuclear power, as an important scientific and technological project, attracts two types of industrial revival that involve the construction of national identity and culture. In the eyes of some government elites, the modernization of nuclear power plants not only underpins the hope of the country's global status of technological prowess, but it is also expected that energy generated endogenously in China will lead to the rise of a new economy. This nuclear power revival gives hopes not only to the thinking of the Chinese rulers, but also to the new expensive nuclear power technology—from reactor to spent fuel disposal—in advanced Western economies. They consider China an overseas test site for such rare technology.

In the 10 years before the Fukushima nuclear accident, the speed and scale of China's nuclear power development rose within a short period. However, because nuclear technology is extremely sensitive, the public raised safety concerns after the Fukushima nuclear accident. The energy security option that once gave hope to nuclear power technology has entered a severe winter, and concerns of development, especially security issues from the perspective of human security, have formed an obstacle to this field (although this sector has been selected for strategic large-scale investment in the Belt and Road Initiative). The policy targets have slowly shown less promise in the latest five-year plan period.

The main reason for the slow development of nuclear power plants after the Fukushima incident was the seemingly sporadic but widespread bottom-up nuclear power resistance activities. The collusion between local governments and central state-owned enterprises in nuclear power development formed after 2005 because a source of local protests that not only affected the economic development planning of a small number of principal officials, but also caused the unpredictable nightmare of social disturbances and mass movements, especially in the eastern coastal areas, often at pre-determined sites for nuclear power plant construction. In many cases, after the information concerning site selection appeared, there was an unpredictable large-scale spontaneous demonstration in an attempt to block the site selection plan.

From the events of Lianyungang, Weihai, Jiangmen, Rushan, and Heshan, we can see that the reasons for the frequent frustration of new nuclear power construction and even the site selection of inland nuclear power plants are to some extent related to the inherent culture of the policy structure and the rigidity of the government's management and governance mentality. Because this is an extremely sensitive topic, policy-makers and business operations often bypass the local residents and rarely deliberate decisions transparently with the discussion of local residents. They often conduct decision-making processes from top to bottom in a habitual and arbitrary way before communicating with stakeholders. However, the starting point for resistance often appears in a (perhaps blindly) confident political culture that seems to be reckless. When top-level decisions of government officials are implemented in local areas, they seldom communicate on development policies and ignore the safety concerns of local residents. Decision-making discussions are often limited to certain circles of specific elite groups. There has been a wave of opposition, albeit sporadic rather than national resistance. The failure of such a series of policy implementations has also hindered the central government's investment in this industry for many years (Toke et al. 2021). Overall, the strategy of diversification of energy options has seemed to complicate the issues relating to both green and human security in a broad sense, which seem difficult to harmonize in the era of environmental precarity.

Electric Vehicles

China's electric vehicle production has increased rapidly in the past few years. With huge growth, in terms of quantity, China has already emerged as the world's largest electric vehicle market. Most owners of new energy vehicles are located in metropolitan areas, where the policy of restricted license exists. Giant cities such as Beijing, Shanghai, Guangzhou, and Shenzhen have become the main growth areas for such new vehicles. The changes in the industrial policy for the growth of automobiles, including preferential measures, have gradually become the core of the analysis and discussion of many researchers. From the general policy framework, we can see that the breakthrough in the development of electric vehicles to some extent is indeed buttressed by local industrial policies under the support of the central government.

To further mitigate the risk of energy insecurity, the 12th Five-Year Guidelines (2010–2015) propose, in terms of investment in green technology, the improvement of internal combustion engine technology and the miniaturization of vehicles as a requirement to reduce fuel consumption as part of the green development of the automotive industry. At the same time, the state proposes that units at all levels promote the application of hybrid technology and develop small pure electric vehicles and plug-in hybrid power. This new policy initiative lays the foundation for the next five years to some extent. In the 13th Five-Year Guidelines (2015–2020), we have seen the government's efforts to improve the power system of vehicles. With increased attention to electrification, Battery-electric vehicles and fuel-cell vehicles have emerged as the main products benefitting from the government's industrial policies during this period, as pointed out in the 12th Five-Year Special Guidelines for the

Development of Electric Vehicle Technology issued by the Ministry of Science and Technology in 2012: "From the perspective of cultivating strategic emerging industries, the development of *pure electric drive* (纯电驱动) electric vehicles with a relatively high degree of electrification is the top priority of development for China's new energy vehicle technology" (Ministry of Science and Technology 2012, 7). However, this type of development strategy emphasizes the driving force of quality promotion. These efforts do not imply that China's climate technology products have established international advantages. In fact, companies still have insufficient investment in research and development. The lack of coordination of the government's multi-headed development has still demonstrated the common problems with the catching-up strategy in the developing world. That is, Chinese automakers are still struggling with the ability to gain a global edge in mid- to high-end technology competition. The pure electric drive platform technology, which is reflected in domestic mid- to high-level and above cars, is not yet mature enough to become a mainstream consumer product.

China's transformation towards a purely electric-driven automobile industry is still in its infancy, although it is obvious that many of these policies are implemented in the effort to reduce oil consumption and CO_2 emissions. The revolution has yet to occur in the auto industry. To some extent, environmental awareness and consumption as a personal reflective lifestyle have not yet become mainstream in China. So far, even though the industrial chain already exists in a rudimentary form, in reality, Chinese policy elites still believe that the electric automobile industry is in a policy market (Lin 2019, 196–197). By investigating policy documents from 2019 to 2020, we can detect changes in political and economic conditions. New energy vehicles were not a policy area that received much attention before 2014. However, since 2015, the industry, as mentioned earlier, has shown momentum in rapid growth. Throughout 2015, China's new production and sales of energy vehicles exceeded 300,000 units, making it the world's largest new energy vehicle market (Xinhua Agency 2016). From 2015 to 2018, the average annual growth rate of China's total production of new energy commercial vehicles, pure electric vehicles, and commercial vehicles and plug-in hybrid commercial vehicles was 18, 25, and 34% respectively. Most of this growth occurred in the pilot cities selected by the central government that include restricted license cities such as Beijing, Shanghai, Guangzhou, Hangzhou, and Tianjin. Furthermore, consumers' car purchase intentions arise from the economic benefits of policy subsidies (Lin 2019, 196–197).

To a certain extent, the motivation for environmental policy is not only the establishment of the mechanism of economic benefits, but also comes from consumption of green car products in the experience of environmental authoritarianism allowed by the special political system in China (Chen and Lees 2018, 2019). Such a policy paradigm also seems to be reflected in the planning context of China's transportation facilities. These related policies have evolved into a policy initiative—the green public transport system policy initiative—to discuss the extent to which top-level design maximizes the possibility of green development in metropolitan areas. Due to the needs of urbanization, it is imperative for the policy elites to consider the materialization of transport infrastructure without dramatically increasing energy consumption and carbon emission. The central government's goal was to enable more than 60% of all Chinese residents to live in towns in 2020 and 70% by 2030 (NEA et al. 2016). These two projected figures, compared with a real-world total of 36% in 2000, represent a sharp increase, which could lead to a potentially negative environmental impact (Albert and Xu 2016). In such a dramatic urbanization process, enabling the green mobility of citizens is the key to successful policy design. Policymakers must take into account the need for more energy consumption, and this need should not be based on the oil industry's established model of high-carbon economic structure, such as the car-petrol capitalism model in advanced economies (Paterson 2007, 111–112).

As one of the global megacities, Shanghai seems to be the first city in China to have successfully established restrictions on the use of motor vehicles to reduce environmental burdens such as energy consumption and air pollution emissions. Early in 1994, Shanghai launched a controversial policy called the "private vehicle license auction system". This system was introduced by the Shanghai Municipal People's Congress, regulated through the *Shanghai Motor Vehicle Management Regulations* (上海市机动车管理条例), through which a market for auctioning licenses was created. The Shanghai municipal government seeks to control the number of cars in a top-down mode by implementing an auction-based license trading market. According to the regulation, the Shanghai municipal government stipulates that both domestic and imported cars are subject to government regulations, and the auction revenue is owned by the state (Han et al. 2014). The state will intervene in the market using suppression measures when the price of a license plate reaches a trigger point. Such measures may include announcing a warning price, which would prohibit bidders from raising their prices any higher, as well as other initiatives to control Shanghai's license market. At the same time, since the central government introduced the Guidance of the State Council on the Priority of the City to Develop Public Transport (State Council 2012b), the Shanghai municipal government has started to reinvest the accumulated revenue of the auction funds for the maintenance or construction of public transport infrastructure, such as rail traffic. The evidence indicates that such initiatives are positive (Darido et al. 2014). Shanghai's policy innovation seems to have become a case of environmental governance policy designed according to what is known as the "polluter pay principle" in the West. Such a top-down policy seeks to compensate for the loss of environmental goods through state intervention in the market and reduces the loss of agency induced by individual economic actors' negligence of the common external cost during the process of rapid urbanization and development.

The Chinese central government has strategized to set affordable public transport as a priority, designing the process of urbanization as the policy elites in the central government introduce what they see as successful policy experiments in the local government. This promulgation process seems to show a recognition of local innovation, spreading it in scale though the national implementation process. This is an important development that seeks to harness the power of local innovation within the overall framework of central command and control.

Immediately following the introduction of the above-mentioned Guidance of the State Council on the Priority of the City to Develop Public Transport,[2] a series of relevant public transport priority initiatives were stipulated nationally. For example, the Ministry of Transport issued its Opinion on Implementation of the Guidance of the State Council on the Priority of the City to Develop Public Transport (Ministry of Transport 2013), the 13th Five-Year Guidelines of Urban Public Transport

[2] As the first central policy documents issued at the highest level since the founding of the People's Republic of China, which considers public transport a priority in its development strategy, the paper proposed that residents in urban areas should include public transport development funds in the public finance system, explicitly putting forth a focus on increasing large-capacity public transport, adding and upgrading the equipment according to local conditions, and seeking corresponding financial capacity to achieve policy goals.

(Ministry of Transport 2016a), and the Guidance of Steady Improvement on the Integration of Urban and Rural Transport to Enhance the Level of Public Service (Ministry of Transport 2016b) issued by 11 central governmental agencies in 2016. In 2017, in the newly introduced 13th Five-Year Guidance of the Development of Modern Integrated Transport System (State Council 2017), the central government further established centralized policy incentives, including a tax exemption for urban bus purchases and exemption from the station land use tax. These policy measures displayed a kind of government-led, market-oriented style of planning to strengthen regulation and political control in the process of new urbanization, with a clear mindset towards top-down unified incentives. At the same time, testing of system implementation has been carried out mutually between local policy experimentation and central implementation. This series of policy measures provides a planning outcome alternative to the orthodox mechanism used in advanced capitalist economies, where policy motivations, outcomes, and the patterns of policy design for the development of urbanization infrastructure are very different than in capitalist states with large territories, such as the United States, Canada, and Australia, where policy models are designed to favour individual vehicle users instead of mass public transport users (Manaugh et al. 2015; Weiner 2016).

The new energy vehicle is a coordinated product under the above-mentioned overall transportation development plan, and it is an auxiliary project of the energy transformation proposed by the central government in recent years. The state aims to gradually carry out industrial transformation through the introduction of industrial policies to promote technological upgrading and even the greening of the automobile industry. To a certain extent, the industrial policy has continued the economic governance of the central government's past desires for cultivating the automobile industry, insisting on a pilot activity emphasizing the learning mechanism of Sino-foreign collaboration and market-for-technology trading. This implies that the government, especially the local government, must actively play the role of planning policy incentives during the industry cultivation period, gather technological and industrial resources, and encourage selected candidates to develop and produce energy-saving and new energy vehicles. In the process of energy transition, the state is required to play the driving role of industrial development, in the sense of a development-oriented economy focused on resource allocation, and to promote the large-scale commercial application of energy saving and new energy vehicles (State Council 2012a). Since 2010, the central government's mindset of development has focused on supporting the new industry. However, compared with other emerging industries, such as non-hydro renewable energy, the role of the state is more diverse and gradual. For new green automobiles, the government first introduced the national new energy vehicle demonstration project to promote applications of new technologies. A unique phenomenon is that compared with the vitality and preferential attention of state-owned enterprises in other fields of science and technology, a more diversified industrial policy guidance method for battery technologies has been achieved. Governments and related enterprises at all levels emphasize diversified development during the construction of charging infrastructure. New market participants are not only large central enterprises, but also include local state-owned enterprises and private enterprises. Foreign-funded enterprises are also gradually participating in the construction of charging infrastructure. In this initial multidimensional policy guidance process, several pilot cities were selected by the central government, such as the charging network in Shenzhen, Hangzhou, Hefei, and other places, gradually forming a large-scale urban charging service network. Furthermore, new innovative technologies such as artificial intelligence applications for traffic management and the informatization and automation of charging infrastructure are gradually emerging. The above descriptions are in line with the planning and development of the National Development and Reform Commission, reflected in policy documents such as the Electric Vehicle Charging Infrastructure Development Guidelines (2015–2020) issued in 2015. In this lengthy and detailed document, the central government's policymakers gave a rough planning idea of how to divide regions, while diversifying economic actors and the participation models of regional and local governments for 2016–2020. It was expected that the country would add more than 7400 centralized charging stations and more than 2.5 million distributed charging stations nationwide to meet the charging needs of more than 2.66 million electric vehicles.

This plan seeks to be compatible with the development of the local area in a manner adapted to local conditions. The government deliberately selects the test sites based on the principal of *youdian zhi mian*—trying to extend the demonstration project from point to surface to the whole country, if it succeeds. The central government arranges targets for these selected locations through digital methods, and the policy targets serve as the basis for giving the carrot and stick of future governance to promote the activities of economic actors. An important figure is the so-called public charging pile-to-electric vehicle ratio. The central government requires this ratio in pilot cities to be no less than 1:7. In other cities, the ratio must strive to reach 1:12. However, to a certain extent, these new governance strategies are mostly limited to large urban areas. Regarding the infrastructure network construction of new energy vehicles, due to smog and public demand, most of the central government priority planning has been located in selected cities in the Beijing-Tianjing-Hebei-Shandong, Yangtze River Delta, and Pearl River Delta regions. This supplementary industrial policy can be said to maintain the existing political and economic structure and gradually increase certain mandatory policy tools in the existing unsustainable policy framework. These policy tools seem to be a nominal environmental policy, but in essence, they are based on a bottom-up decision model that no longer depends on emancipatory autonomous environmental politics but is more inclined to expand expert-based policy bureaucratic decisions. That said, I contend that that the new vehicle industries are not positioned as strategic industries, so the economic structure's advantage level provides leeway and discretionary powers that enable local governments to create such policy markets. Balancing excessive protection and innovation drivers is the ultimate key to accelerating the production and diffusion of hydrogen and fuel-cell technologies.

Discussion and Conclusion

Comparing the nuclear power and non-hydro renewable energy development systems, one point that few observers mentioned is that, to some extent, although both are formed under the hierarchical system of China's public governance system, non-hydro renewable energy seems to have shown relatively successful development results in the control of a centralized governing structure. This success includes the cultivation of domestic industrial manufacturing, export activity, output value, and, more importantly, the quantity and quality of technological innovation. In contrast, nuclear power plant development seems to have gradually lost its comparative advantage in the mixed energy policy options through the long process of the government's industrial cultivation. To some extent, this lies in the human security issues that are rooted in specific energy choices for development. Compared with traditional fuel choices, wind power and solar power are less hindered by conventional utilities when they are promoted. This has been a relatively easy policy result in the central government's decision. Unlike coal, the policy arena often involves provision of labour employment and local governments' interest entanglements and even corruption. Furthermore, hydroelectric power also affects large-scale migration and degradation of natural resources and other non-traditional security concerns.

Nuclear power seems to have a broader scope. As a specific energy source that may cause endogenous non-traditional security (Xiao 2019, 52), to some extent, after the Fukushima incident in Japan, it seems to have instantly become a source of social disagreement among citizens. Considered a potential source of chaos, most of the originally planned nuclear power projects were either suspended or delayed in delivery. For example, the new third-generation reactor unit of nuclear power in cooperation with France was delayed for many years. Although there have been years of Sino-foreign cooperation and exchanges in nuclear power plant construction, it seems that only the local units of Hualong No. 1 have been able to make steady progress in numerous nuclear power development and innovation projects. It is not difficult to see that COVID-19 has drastically delayed the economic development of and political actors' ambition for nuclear power plant deployment meeting the policy installation targets set forth in the 13th Five-Year Plan.

More and more political discourse began to revolve around so-called people-based discussions. However, the paradox is that this new explanation of human security has been promoted in political issues with the establishment of the central government's new apparatus, the National Security Commission (NSC). On the one hand, the government emphasizes a diverse and universal security concept, advocating the highest security concept of the so-called "community with a shared future for mankind (*renlei mingyun gongtong ti*)". On the other hand, the government elites claim that this is a diverse, non-state-centric security concept that can coexist with the traditional state-based security involving sovereignty issues. Among them, in terms of issues related to the earth system, are energy poverty, environmental degradation, and proposing a more sustainably benign economic development model. To some extent, these narratives are contained in a relatively new political discourse, namely "building a harmonious society" and the so-called security concept that refocuses on the quality of development, economic development, and the quality of life of the masses.

The paradox is that considering the multifaceted nature of nuclear power plants and the potential social and technical risks, it is difficult to resolve the dilemma and contradiction between the perceived context and the concerns of the local people through the amendment of narratives alone. It seems difficult to generalize discourses surrounding nuclear power plants that are easily classified as "clean energy" with an expectation of neutralizing the risks. The discourse constructed in layers still seems to be unable to change the long-standing attitude and resistance of residents. To some extent, it has formed a kind of institutional problem amidst the global pandemic. Under COVID-19 where internal and external safety concerns are tense, nuclear power plants (considering the lack of solutions for the storage and processing of nuclear spent fuels so far) and the risks in the contemporary security narrative have indeed introduced alternative instability factors to the so-called new thinking of governing for the people, and at the same time, it is difficult to satisfy the need of human security in the era of global warming. The current local challenges involving human security issues may not lie in the rise and fall of solar, wind, or nuclear power plants under the spotlight. For policymakers, a more acute challenge is the energy supply in rural areas. To date, a number of rural residents in China still do not have the living support of the modern power system and proper access to energy. Most of the energy they use comes from the traditional method of biomass energy, which is the burning of straw, although in recent years, commercial power generation has gradually supplied rural electrification.

Beginning in 2003, the central government invested and built power grid infrastructure, focusing on rural areas. Certain specific policies have been introduced, along with the strategy of the plan of Western Development (*Xibu da kaifa*), such as the "Brightness Programme" and "Township Electrification Programme". This policy scheme aims to help people in rural areas generate electricity through renewable energy equipment in an off-grid environment. The "Township Electrification Programme", as another auxiliary policy measure, also provides cost subsidies for power generation equipment to users in western regions such as Qinghai, Xinjiang, Inner Mongolia, Shaanxi, Sichuan, and Tibet (Han et al. 2014, 230). These regional development strategies, which have been continuously emphasized by administrations from Hu-Wen to Xi-Li, are to a considerable extent through the central government's regulatory intervention to solve the problem of energy poverty while meeting (although restricted to the sense of economic development) human security requirements. Following the COVID-19 situation, the government's effectiveness and the role of the central state seem to have increasingly become more significant, in both narrative and practice. Local governments' autonomy may not be temporarily reinvigorated following the COVID-19 situation, especially considering the central government once dispatched its authority to curb the national epidemic. Under the continued challenges of the next economic development, it is likely that the long-term issue of energy security via transition to new energy will be extended due to the unexpected epidemic, and it may not be regarded as an urgent crisis at this stage. The priority of the policy position of environmental security may be sacrificed briefly. The powerful motivation behind the imperative of the green economy has always been a complementary element to the catching-up mindset of economic development. In the end, the key to the success of ensuring energy security lies in the extent to which one can form a truly organic connection between national security and human security in the Chinese context.

References

Albert, Eleanor, and Beina Xu. 2016. 'China's Environmental Crisis'. CFR Backgrounders. Available at http://www.cfr.org/china/chinas-environmental-crisis/p12608 (accessed 18 November 2020).

Andrews-Speed, Philip. 2020. 'China's Efforts to Constrain Its Fossil Fuel Consumption'. In *The Palgrave Handbook of Managing Fossil Fuels and Energy Transitions*, edited by Geoffrey Wood and Keith Baker, 109–37. Cham: Springer International Publishing. https://doi.org/10.1007/978-3-030-28076-5_5.

Blühdorn, Ingolfur. 2020. 'The Legitimation Crisis of Democracy: Emancipatory Politics, the Environmental State and the Glass Ceiling to Socio-Ecological Transformation'. *Environmental Politics* 29 (1): 38–57.

Callahan, William A. 2012. 'China's Strategic Futures: Debating the Post-American World Order'. *Asian Survey* 52 (4): 617–42. https://doi.org/10.1525/as.2012.52.4.617.

Chen, Geoffrey C., and Charles Lees. 2016. 'Growing China's Renewables Sector: A Developmental State Approach'. *New Political Economy* 21 (6): 574–86. https://doi.org/10.1080/13563467.2016.1183113.

———. 2018. 'The New, Green, Urbanization in China: Between Authoritarian Environmentalism and Decentralization'. *Chinese Political Science Review*, February, 1–20. https://doi.org/10.1007/s41111-018-0095-1.

———. 2019. 'Political Recentralisation and the Diffusion of Solar Energy in China'. *Europe-Asia Studies* 71 (7): 1162–82. https://doi.org/10.1080/09668136.2019.1619669.

———. 2021. 'Greening the Chinese Leviathan: China's Renewable Energy Governance as a Source of Soft Power.' *Journal of International Relations and Development*. https://doi.org/10.1057/s41268-021-00213-3.

Chen, Zhiting, and Geoffrey C. Chen. 2019. 'The Changing Political Economy of Central State-Owned Oil Companies in China'. *The Pacific Review* 34 (3): 379–404.

'China's Energy Policy: New Technology and Civil Nuclear Expansion'. 2016. *Strategic Comments* 22 (1): vii–viii. https://doi.org/10.1080/13567888.2016.1170408.

China Southern Power Grid. 2019. '2019 China Southern Power Grid Renewable Energy Development Report [2019 年中国南方电网可再生能源发展报告]'. Beijing: China Electric Power Press.

Dannreuther, Roland. 2017. *Energy Security*. Cambridge: Polity Press.

Darido, Georges, Torresmontoya, Mariana, and Mehndiratta, Shomik Raj. 2014. 'Urban Transport and CO2 Emissions: Some Evidence from Chinese Cities'. *Wiley Interdisciplinary Reviews: Energy and Environment* 3 (2): 122–55.

Ding, Ming, Zhicheng Xu, Weisheng Wang, Xiuli Wang, Yunting Song, and Dezhi Chen. 2016. 'A Review on China's Large-Scale PV Integration: Progress, Challenges and Recommendations'. *Renewable and Sustainable Energy Reviews* 53 (January): 639–52. https://doi.org/10.1016/j.rser.2015.09.009.

Economy, Elizabeth C. 2018. *The Third Revolution: Xi Jinping and the New Chinese State*. Oxford: Oxford University Press.

Forrest, Robert, and Chaim Braun. 2017. 'Managing China's Spent Nuclear Fuel: A Model Framework for Interim Storage'. *The Nonproliferation Review* 24 (1–2): 31–45. https://doi.org/10.1080/10736700.2017.1385732.

Foster, Emma. 2013. 'Green Security'. In *Critical Approaches to Security: An Introduction to Theories and Methods*, edited by Laura J. Shepherd, 37–50. Abingdon: Routledge.

Gao, Baiyu. 2020. 'Despite coronavirus, China Aims for Renewables Grid Parity.' *China Dialogue*, 2 June. https://chinadialogue.net/en/energy/despite-coronavirus-china-aims-for-renewables-grid-parity/. Accesssed 27 August 2020.

Global Energy Interconnection Development and Cooperation Organization (GEIDCO). 2020. 'Research on China's Energy Reform and Transformation based on the New Development Concept [新发展理念的中国能源变

革转型研究]'. https://www.geidco.org/html/qqnyhlw/zt20200731/index.html#research. Accessed 20 August 2020.

Gosens, Jorrit, and Frank Jotzo. 2020. 'China's Post-COVID-19 Stimulus: No Green New Deal in Sight'. *Environmental Innovation and Societal Transitions* 36 (September): 250–54. https://doi.org/10.1016/j.eist.2020.07.004.

Gosens, Jorrit, and Yonglong Lu. 2014. 'Prospects for Global Market Expansion of China's Wind Turbine Manufacturing Industry'. *Energy Policy* 67 (April): 301–18. https://doi.org/10.1016/j.enpol.2013.12.055.

Han, Shu, Zhang, Hua, and Chen, Xiaohong. 2014. 'Intervention Policies for Private Car Ownership in Megacities of Developing Countries'. *Transportation Research Record: Journal of the Transportation Research Board* 2451: 68–76.

Han, Wenke, Luo, Zhihong, and Fan Lijuan. 2014. 'Striving towards Development: China's Efforts to Alleviate Energy Poverty'. In *Energy Poverty: Global Challenges and Local Solutions*, edited by Antoine Halff, Benjamin K. Sovacool, and Jon Rozhon, 225–236. Oxford: Oxford University Press.

Hochstetler, Kathryn, and Genia Kostka. 2015. 'Wind and Solar Power in Brazil and China: Interests, State–Business Relations, and Policy Outcomes'. *Global Environmental Politics* 15 (3): 74–94. https://doi.org/10.1162/GLEP_a_00312.

Hudson, Natalie Florea, Alex Kreidenweis, and Charli Carpenter. 2013. 'Human Security'. In *Critical Approaches to Security: An Introduction to Theories and Methods*, edited by Laura J. Shepherd, 24–36. Abingdon: Routledge.

Kirkegaard, Julia Kirch. 2019. *Wind Power in China: Ambiguous Winds of Change in China's Energy Market* Abingdon: Routledge.

Lewis, Joanna. 2007. 'Technology Acquisition and Innovation in the Developing World: Wind Turbine Development in China and India'. *Studies in Comparative International Development (SCID)* 42 (3): 208–32. https://doi.org/10.1007/s12116-007-9012-6.

Lin, Boqiang. 2019. 'China Energy Outlook 2019 [中国能源发展报告 2019]'. Beijing: Peking University Press.

Manaugh, Kevin, Badami, Madhav G., and Ahmed M. El-Geneidy. 2015. 'Integrating Social Equity into Urban Transportation Planning: A Critical Evaluation of Equity Objectives and Measures in Transportation Plans in North America'. *Transport Policy* 37: 167–76.

Marks, D. 2010. 'China's Climate Change Policy Process: Improved but Still Weak and Fragmented'. *Journal of Contemporary China* 19 (67): 971–86.

Mathews, John A., and Hao Tan. 2014. 'Energy: China Leads the Way on Renewables'. *Nature* 508 (7496): 319–19. https://doi.org/10.1038/508319a.

———. 2015. *China's Renewable Energy Revolution*. Palgrave Macmillan. http://www.palgraveconnect.com/doifinder/10.1057/9781137546258.

McNally, Amy, Darrin Magee, and Aaron T. Wolf. 2009. 'Hydropower and Sustainability: Resilience and Vulnerability in China's Powersheds'. *Journal of Environmental Management*, Understanding and Linking the Biophysical, Socio Economic and Geopolitical Effects of Dams 90 (July): S286–93. https://doi.org/10.1016/j.jenvman.2008.07.029.

Ministry of Science and Technology. 2012. 'Notice on Printing and Distributing the "Twelfth Five-Year" Special Plan for the Development of Electric Vehicle Technology [关于印发电动汽车科技发展"十二五"专项规划的通知]'. *Guokefaji*, 195.

Ministry of Transport. 2013. 'Opinion on Implementation of the Guidance of the State Council on the Priority of the City to Develop Public Transport [交通运输部关于贯彻落实《国务院关于城市优先发展公共交通的指导意见》的实施意见]'. *Jiaoyunfa*, 368.

Ministry of Transport. 2016a. 'The Thirteen Five-Year Guidelines of Urban Public Transport [交通运输部关于印发《城市公共交通"十三五"发展纲要》的通知]'. 18 July. http://www.gov.cn/xinwen/2016-07/25/content_5094575.htm Accessed 20 December 2020.

Ministry of Transport. 2016b. 'The Guidance of Steady Improvement on the Integration of Urban and Rural Transport to Enhance the Level of Public Service [关于稳步推进城乡交通运输一体化提升公共服务水平的指导意见]'. *Jiaoyunfa*, 184.

Nahm, Jonas. 2017. 'Exploiting the Implementation Gap: Policy Divergence and Industrial Upgrading in China's Wind and Solar Sectors'. *The China Quarterly*, August, 1–23. https://doi.org/10.1017/S030574101700090X.

Nahm, Jonas, and Edward S. Steinfeld. 2014. 'Scale-Up Nation: China's Specialization in Innovative Manufacturing'. *World Development* 54 (February): 288–300. https://doi.org/10.1016/j.worlddev.2013.09.003.

National Energy Administration (NEA), Development Research Center of the State Council (DRCSC), and Ministry of Land and Resources of the PRC. 2016. 'China Natural Gas Development Report 2016 [中国天然气发展报告2016]'. Beijing: Petroleum Industry Press.

Nyman, Jonna. 2016. 'What is the Value of Security? Contextualising the Negative/Positive Debate'. *Review of International Studies* 42 (5): 821–839.

Nyman, Jonna. 2018. *The Energy Security Paradox: Rethinking Energy (in)Security in the United States and China*. Oxford University Press.

Nyman, Jonna and Jinghan Zeng. 2016. 'Securitization in Chinese Climate and Energy Politics'. *WIREs Climate Change* 7: 301–313.

Paterson, Mathew. 2007. *Automobile Politic: Ecology and Cultural Political Economy*. Cambridge: Cambridge University Press.

Pelenc, Jérôme, and Dubois, Jean-Luc. 2020. 'Human Development and Strong Sustainability: A Mutual Dialogue.' In *Sustainability, Capabilities and Human Security*, edited by Andrew Crabtree, 19–50. Cham: Palgrave Macmillan.

Qi, Ye, Wenjuan Dong, Changgui Dong, and Caiwei Huang. 2019. 'Understanding Institutional Barriers for Wind Curtailment in China'. *Renewable and Sustainable Energy Reviews* 105 (May): 476–86. https://doi.org/10.1016/j.rser.2019.01.061.

REN21. 2019. *Renewables 2019 Global Status Report*. Paris: REN21 Secretariat.

Shapiro, Judith. 2012. *China's Environmental Challenges*. Cambridge: Polity Press.

State Council. 2012a. 'Development Guidance of Energy-saving and New Energy Automobile Industry (2012–2020) [节能与新能源汽车产业发展规划] (2012-2020年))'. Guofa No. 22.

State Council. 2012b. 'The Guidance of the State Council on the Priority of the City to Develop Public Transport [国务院关于城市优先发展公共交通的指导意见]'. 29 December. Guofa No. 64.

State Council. 2017. 'The Development Guidance of the Thirteenth Five-Year Modern Integrated Transport System [十三五"现代综合交通运输体系发展规划]'. Guofa No. 11.

Statista. 2020. 'Volume of Nuclear Energy Produced and Connected to the Grid in China from 2009 to 2019 (in Billion Kilowatthours)'. *China Dialogue*. Available at: https://www.statista.com/statistics/1202983/china-volume-of-nuclear-energy-generatedand-connected-to-the-grid/. Accessed 31 August 2021.

Thomson, Elspeth. 2011. 'China's Nuclear Energy in Light of the Disaster in Japan'. *Eurasian Geography and Economics* 52 (4): 464–82. https://doi.org/10.2747/1539-7216.52.4.464.

Toke, David. 2017. *China's Role in Reducing Carbon Emissions: The Stabilisation of Energy Consumption and the Deployment of Renewable Energy*.

Toke, David, Geoffrey Chun-fung Chen, Antony Froggatt, and Richard Connolly. 2021. *Nuclear Power in Stagnation: A Cultural Approach to Failed Expansion*. Abingdon: Routledge.

Weiner, Edward. 2016. *Urban Transportation Planning In The United States: History, Policy, and Practice* (5th ed). Switzerland: Springer.

Xiao, Ren. 2019. 'Human Security in Practice: The Chinese Experience'. In *Human Security Norms in East Asia*, edited by Yoichi Mine, Oscar A. Gómez, and Ako Muto. Cham: Palgrave Macmillan.

Xinhua Agency. 2016. 'Vice Minister of Industry and Information Technology: There is Still a Big Gap Between the Quality of China's New Energy Vehicles and the World's Advanced Level [工信部副部长: 我国新能源汽车品质与世界先进水平还有较大差距]', 23 January. https://business.sohu.com/20160123/n435618533.shtml. Accessed 25 December 2020.

Yip, George S., and Bruce McKern. 2016. *China's Next Strategic Advantage: From Imitation to Innovation*. http://lib.myilibrary.com?id=913441.

Zhang, Hui. 2015. 'Uranium Supplies: A Hitch to China's Nuclear Energy Plans? Or Not?' *Bulletin of the Atomic Scientists* 71 (3): 58–66. https://doi.org/10.1177/0096340215581358.

Zhang, Sufang, Philip Andrews-Speed, and Sitao Li. 2018. 'To What Extent Will China's Ongoing Electricity Market Reforms Assist the Integration of Renewable Energy?' *Energy Policy* 114 (March): 165–72. https://doi.org/10.1016/j.enpol.2017.12.002.

Zhou, Yun. 2011. 'China's Spent Nuclear Fuel Management: Current Practices and Future Strategies'. *Energy Policy*, Special Section: Renewable Energy Policy and Development 39 (7): 4360–69. https://doi.org/10.1016/j.enpol.2011.04.055.

Zhu, Mengye, Ye Qi, David Belis, Jiaqi Lu, and Bart Kerremans. 2019. 'The China Wind Paradox: The Role of State-Owned Enterprises in Wind Power Investment Versus Wind Curtailment'. *Energy Policy* 127 (April): 200–12. https://doi.org/10.1016/j.enpol.2018.10.059.

Zhang, Hui. 2015. Uranium Supplies: A Hitch to China's Nuclear Energy Plans? … [illegible]

[illegible]

[illegible]

[illegible]

CHAPTER 5

The Education for Patriotism in Post-Pandemic China: The CCP's Approach to "Psychological Insecurity" in Focus

Jinru Huang

Introduction

As covid-19 sweeps the globe, the term "Chinese virus" pervades and is strongly defended in Western social media. While other countries are suffering from their first wave, China has begun to revive from paralyses due to the alleged superiorities of political institution and leadership. Facing racist and McCarthyistic comments, and charges of being a public health superpower in funding the complicit relation with the WHO and not being transparent enough, Beijing retaliates by propagating its successes and other country's setbacks to provoke patriotism and national identification domestically.

This chapter is written in the context of a global pandemic that witnesses a new wave of patriotic education launched in China. The covid-19 pandemic has been generating new discourses of Chinese nationalism

J. Huang (✉)
University of Leeds, Leeds, UK
e-mail: pt17j3h@leeds.ac.uk

C. Zhang (ed.), *Human Security in China*,
https://doi.org/10.1007/978-981-16-4675-1_5

in response to anti-Chinese sentiments and presenting new challenges to the political legitimacy of the party-state, in which cases the school as the battlefield of one's political socialisation is held accountable to foster favourable orientation and subjectivity and to wipe off "ideological pollution". In this context, patriotic education plays a key role in mobilising Chinese students against "Western conspiracy" and "hostile ideology" that permeate schools upon reopening.

This chapter examines the construction of "psychological security" as part of the human security "with Chinese characteristics". In response to the security threats that came from foreign hostilities, patriotic education has contributed to breeding and reproducing Chinese nationalism amongst Chinese students. The education for patriotism has strengthened students' identification with the "socialist cause" and instilled confidence in the Chinese Communist Party (CCP) leadership of the Chinese youth by using epistemologically constructed sources of security to dispel "psychological insecurity" at home. This chapter contributes to the record of the development of China's ideological indoctrination during the pandemic and provides a seasonable check on the securitisation of the interference in the people's psychological security building in post-pandemic China.

Reconceptualising Human Security in the Chinese Context

It is impossible and insufficient to study Chinese politics without considering the centrality of the Chinese Communist Party (CCP) in this party-state. In July 2021, the CCP celebrated its centenary, when slogans that have been popular for years, such as "without the Communist Party, there would be no new China," were once again chanted throughout the country. At this time, learning the history of the Party has become the focus of a new round of political work within the CCP as well as in government, military, and all other public sector agencies in China.

On this occasion, CCP put two things in the spotlight for the nation to celebrate: one is the eradication of poverty—the CCP announced its success in lifting almost 100 million Chinese people out of poverty that had plagued it for so long before the centenary of the founding of the CCP; the other is an answer sheet of near perfection in responding to the global pandemic on the battlefield in China. The commonality to both of the above is that they are achieved under the CCP leadership and they are two of the most significant successes of recent years that underpin the regime's legitimacy. These attempts and achievements have not only paved the way for the Chinese President Xi Jinping's claim to absolute personal authority at CCP's 12th National Congress and shaped the Party's image as the pushing hand that has led China ever closer to the great rejuvenation of the Chinese nation, but also brought enough sense of security to the people and made them believe that they live in a country that is sufficiently strong and safe.

Unlike "Western" perceptions of human security which often associate security with human needs and human rights in the broadest sense[1] and the emphasis on the shared responsibility of all countries to intervene and protect, China tends to be wary of using this foreign term in avoiding excessive empowerment of individual rights and maintaining the status quo that national sovereignty takes precedence over individual rights in many cases. China is cautious about adopting the aforementioned concept of human security because blindly embracing a concept that may be incompatible with the existing regime is viewed as potentially subversive.

On the one hand, human security, as is understood by the international community, is more or less relevant to state-to-state relations. For more than half a century the Chinese diplomacy has been guided by an independent foreign policy of peace,[2] in which the principles do not involve interference in recognising the threats to human security and the approaches to be taken to safeguard that security of other countries. And vice versa, Beijing does not expect any outside interference in its diagnosis of the factors that threaten its domestic human security. On the other hand, China appears to be able to justify that national sovereignty must at some point precede human security. From the public's point of view, there seems to be a certain consensus in China that the latter is a prerequisite for the former.

[1] See *Human Development Report* (UNDP 1994) which identifies human security through seven categories, including economic, food, health, environmental, personal, community/identity and political (freedoms) security.

[2] Known as the Five Principles of Peaceful Coexistence: mutual respect for sovereignty and territorial integrity, mutual non-aggression, non-interference in each other's internal affairs, equality and mutual benefit, and peaceful coexistence, first codified in 1954 and stated in the Sino-Indian Agreement.

However, the CCP's understanding of human security is different. Whether it is the experience of having been invaded by the foreign powers in modern history or the most recent covid-19 thought to have originated in China and then fast spread the globe that stirs up another wave of anti-China sentiments, the greatest lesson that the Chinese people have been taught is that the security of the Chinese people must not rely on foreign countries but its own state. As thus, the human security definition and agenda in China have often held hostage to a spirit of dedication and sacrifice that anchored in collectivism, which glorifies the feat of individual sacrifice for the good of the whole and has led to a less human-centred discourse on human security in China. While on the contrary, the CCP's version of human security is more akin to paternalistic concerns for both ideological and biopolitical security of the Chinese people as a collective which, for sure, merely humanises the existing discourse for state security.

In addition, China's obsession with collectivism must be factored into the analysis of the country's interpretation of and agenda for human security. As distinct from the state-individual security tension, there is another in-between consideration of *communities* that shall be taken into account. The antipathy and discrimination triggered by the pandemic can be found everywhere around the world. Yet, in China, the changing relations between the state, communities and individuals deserve some serious reflections. Notable examples of these changing relations are how Wuhanese and the Chinese overseas students have been asked by their fellow citizens for extra levels of "sacrifice". For instance, the willingness to cooperate with the government in staying inside of the city during a months-long municipal lockdown, or choosing not to increase the government's burden by staying outside the country when imported covid cases were reported to be largely the students studying abroad. These cases suggest that as lockdowns rolled out, communities began to take on the role of policing individuals and link the sacrifice of the latter to patriotism. Thus, communities contributed to increased tensions between state security and the security of individuals. The pandemic highlights the zero-sum mentality of human security in the Chinese context—the security of "human" as a collective is deemed only achievable with the sacrifices of the security of "human" as individuals.

Therefore, weighing gains and losses is the regular topic in safeguarding the "greater good" which invariably involves the government to guide communities to help the state justify its security priority and agenda. The regime's legitimacy that is supposed to be obtained by ensuring the security of each individual has been relaxed its standards by defining the scope of the collective and looking after the vast majority's interest rather than that of those who may be in the depths of despair. It can be seen that the political wisdom of the CCP to "unite the greatest possible forces" is still evident in human security issues arising from the pandemic. By protecting the collective defined by it and ignoring the antagonism perceived between the collective and certain communities, the CCP has been able to continue to benefit from political stability and state security.

Given the above, studying the essence and approach of human security in China must not be based on the conventional nor Western human security perceptions and narratives solely for value judgements, but requires developing the manifestation and significance of human security in the Chinese context while building on the conventional perspectives. In this way, not only does such re-contextualisation correspond to the trends among many human security analysts in recent years that human security should be more inclusive of non-traditional security studies in making the notion of human security more accommodative, but it also provides the conceptual premise for the subsequent discussion.

Contextualising School Education for Human Security

Education is often seen as one of the most basic human needs in human security narratives. In the traditional sense, prioritising access to education acknowledges individuals' right to development and helps improve one's life chances. Even though individual capabilities and diligence may be different, education undoubtedly equips learners with skills and credentials (despite its inherently exploitative nature as cultural capital), which secure them in living their economic, cultural, and political lives towards the enhancement of human freedom and capability in general.

However, this observation (of education on human security) is largely based on the idea that the concept of human security is integrally connected with materially securing human capability to develop. Whereas psychological security, or the individual's non-material needs to be in a safe and stable environment in which they can thrive, is equally important. As former US President Roosevelt rightly puts it, '[n]ecessitous men are not free men'.[3] Rather than simply freeing people from the distresses caused by illiteracy and innumeracy,[4] education ought to play a more functional role in eradicating human insecurity caused by uncertainty and instability. This is never an endorsement that justifies any biassed information or predetermined conclusion (e.g. ideological education) should be conveyed or drawn in school. Instead, one should note that the identity of a person and psychological security can and certainly be created and acquired through school education.

In explaining how schools cater to the psychological dimension of human security in an organised and large-scale manner, Lemke's (Lemke 2011) volume on biopolitics can help us understand the special position of schools when it comes to producing "subjects":

> ...subjectivation, that is, the manner in which subjects are brought to work on themselves, guided by...authorities and on the basis of socially accepted arrangements.... How are people called on, in the name of (individual and collective) life and health (one's own health and that of the family, nation...), in view of defined goals to act in a certain way (in extreme cases even to die for such goal)? How are they brought to experience their life as "worthy" or "not worthy" of being lived? How are they interpellated as members of a "higher" or "inferior" race, a "strong" or a "weak" sex, a "rising" or a "degenerate" people?

Lemke's point about students as subjects being made in schools in very different and particular ways is epistemologically constructivist, which is based on the assumption that societal standards of values that affect the direction of the subjectivation of students are socially constructed.[5]

[3] Freedom from Want: From *A Study Guide To The Four Freedoms*, Carnegie Council for Ethics in International Affairs. Accessed on 11 May 2021. Available at: https://www.carnegiecouncil.org/education/001/four_freedoms/5226.

[4] Illiteracy and innumeracy are seen to contribute to sources of insecurity such as unemployment, inability or disfunction to understand and invoke one's legal rights, and constraint to voice one's political views. For women in especial, they are variables for gender inequality. See Sen (2002).

[5] According to Guba and Lincoln (1994) constructivism is a paradigm that promotes unique ontological and epistemological alignment. *Most constructivists would align with a subjective epistemology in which "knowledge is symbolically constructed and understandings of the world are based on conventions* (Hatch 2002, p. 15).

As thus, education is necessarily stratified, as it is perceived to be critically failed to provide an adequate underpinning for free social mobility[6]; rather, schools play the role of "sifting and sorting" agents to ensure meritocracy by preparing the right people to enter the most appropriate jobs and roles in life.[7,8] To do this, in Saltman's (2018) analysis, students are taught in school that their lives are supposed to go in particular directions, and that the luck they have, good or bad, has more to do with their own alleged natural abilities than with the social structures.

By combining the above functionalist and Marxist ideas on education it is crystal clear that education often serves for predetermined formation and cultivation of not only students' academic knowledge and professional skills but also their favourable disposition and ideological instillation that in line with the norms and values of society. This is very true and will be soon analysed in the subsequent section on the Chinese state education system. Yet, based on Lemke's epistemological standpoint that many of the criteria on the norms and values of students are constructed socio-economically and the fact that students are taught and trained differently is very much intertwined with taking certain directions and developing specific ideology in their lives. Taken in this sense, even though education stratifies and exploits, it is more of convergence rather than divergence in terms of unifying thoughts and norms for the sustainability of the social system.

However, what is the connection between the above and human security? If one applies a deconstructive lens over the above discussion, it can be seen that students can also be taught and trained to move in the same direction, or even not to move towards any direction. Accordingly, our understanding of education must not be confined to the perception of sheerly transmitting knowledge and skills. The foregoing consideration suggests that an education that unifies ideas and social

[6] See Bourdieu on social and cultural reproduction (Bourdieu and Passeron 1990).

[7] See Talcott Parsons on functionalism and education. According to Parsons (2008), education helps facilitates role allocation, and the education system helps society to be meritocratic. Whereas Marxist analysts Bowles and Gintis argue that school prepares workers for a life of exploitation in capitalism and reproduces social class inequalities.

[8] For example, see Shavit and Müller (2006) on vocational education and embedded racial inequalities and gender bias inside and outside classroom. See Brown (2018) explanation of education inequality and the "new vocationalism" for inequality both politically and in the classroom.

norms satisfies the psychological security of attendees, whereas uncertainty, instability, and disorder as the source of "psychological insecurity" stemming from disunified thoughts and inconsistent social norms can greatly threaten other dimensions of human security. The significance of education in "psycurely" (psychological-securely) installing students in the given social conditions and (re)producing prescribed ideologies, values and dispositions is therefore discerned in this chapter.

Measuring Psychological Insecurity: Sources and the Nationalist Response in China

Since December 2019, when a novel coronavirus was first found and identified in Wuhan, the hostility against China and the Chinese people has emerged and has been with the entire course of the global pandemic outbreak. Despite swift and serious measures taken by the Chinese government, the ineffectiveness in containing the spread of the virus to the Western world has given the latter a reason to blame the CCP. It has been observed that the covid-19 outbreak has triggered widespread Sinophobic sentiments and behaviours both online and in real life. An increasing spread of Sinophobic content across social media platforms is noted, as demonstrated by blaming China for the situation and using more and new verbal slurs (Tahmasbi et al. 2020; Lee and Li 2021). For offline, the virus-fuelled racial hatred and various forms of discrimination such as verbal abuse, physical attacks, and vandalism have also aroused wide attention in intellectual circles (Coates 2020; Li and Nicholson 2021).

The globally pervasive Sinophobia and racist violence have confused the people in China where the virus had originally hit the hardest. In this case, the psychological effects of the covid-19 pandemic are twofold. Apart from traumatic experiences such as losing loved ones and experiencing fear from food and resource scarcity, there is also psychological distress exacerbated by Sinophobic and anti-Chinese sentiments, stigma and discrimination. Drawing on experience during the peak and long-term recovery from SARS (Misra et al. 2020) argue that anticipating and undergoing race-based discrimination can profoundly affect and increase the risk of mental health problems, causing greater anxiety and uncertainty both amid and after covid-19. As thus, people in China (and potentially other Asian communities) have to cope not only with the impact of the virus itself, but also the *psychological insecurity* surged by racial and cultural stigma as well as the politicisation of this public health crisis.

The covid-19 emergency has sharpened the confrontation between China and the West. It is quite clear that due to narrative spin, agendas, and misinformation, where the virus came from is no longer a scientific question. Instead, it has become a highly politicised debate on the international stage. As observed, politicians were able to drive buzz online, for example, the number of coronavirus-related tweets with anti-Asian hashtags rose dramatically after the former US President Trump tweeted about "the Chinese Virus" (Hswen et al. 2021). Others, such as the governor of the Veneto region of Italy[9] and Brazil's education minister[10] who respectively ridiculed the Chinese people for "eat[ing] mice alive" and suggested covid-19 is part of China's geopolitical plan, have exacerbated racism, misunderstanding, Sinophobia, and anti-Chinese rhetoric. The covid-19 crisis has been maliciously exploited by many Western political parties and groups to promote anti-immigrant, white supremacist, ultra-nationalist, xenophobic conspiracy theories that demonise refugees, foreigners, prominent figures, and political leaders.[11]

On the other side, as will be discussed shortly thereafter, China's response to the rise of Sinophobia and racism has also been politicised. For instance, in the debate over the source of the virus, the spokesman of China's Foreign Ministry Zhao Lijian took the lead in questioning that the US military may have brought covid-19 into Wuhan.[12] As the outbreak had progressed the number of confirmed covid cases outside China outstripped that in China, there was a flurry of opinions on Chinese social media retorted and struck back the offensive racist rhetoric against the Chinese came forth in the early days of the outbreak. The authority seemed to relish Chinese netizens' patriotism in defending the country's image—not only did they acquiesce in the war of words on social media

[9] Extracted from a 2020 Human Right Watch report. Available from: www.hrw.org/news/2020/05/12/covid-19-fueling-anti-asian-racism-and-xenophobia-worldwide.

[10] Ibid.

[11] Ibid.

[12] Zhao (2020) said on his verified Twitter account that the United States was to blame for a lack of transparency about the outbreak, alluded that covid-19 was mistaken for the flu.

platforms, after months of national lockdown and with the pandemic being effectively under control at home, the authority also exploited the outbreak in other countries for propaganda purposes.

As the number of confirmed cases in China continues to fall, articles that praise the "Chinese model" are found abound in official media and online public opinion. The most famous of these was the publication of *China Combating COVID-19 in 2020*, a book published at a time when Wuhan still suffered from huge uncertainty and compiled to praise the leadership and the superiority of China's socialist system. While advocating patriotism in the face of the coronavirus, some official media commentaries seemed to play down, intentionally or not, the response of other countries to covid-19. The *Global Times*, a subsidiary newspaper under the CCP's propaganda flagship the *People's Daily*, published an editorial headlined "Some countries slow to respond to virus" on both its Chinese and English websites (Global Times 2020; Huanqiu Shibao 2020). While pointing out the seriousness of the covid-19 outbreak in Japan, South Korea, Iran and Italy, the article also revealed a "thankfulness" for the Chinese model against covid-19 and a "good luck" to be born in China.

With the emergence of this trend of thinking, some Chinese netizens have called in a playful tone for countries with more modest preventive and control measures to follow the Chinese model, for example by using the expression "do not know to copy and paste China's homework" to satirise countries that are perceived to be incompetent and slow to react in the face of covid-19. It seems that China's response to the sense of insecurity caused by the aforesaid Sinophobic sentiments and inflammatory reactions through portraying its own efforts at home in comparison to other countries' "failure" to prevent the virus from wildly spreading has succeeded in igniting a patriotic fervour in many. Clearly to a large extent the politicisation of public health crisis coupled with a war of propaganda has had a good curative effect in boosting the public's confidence in the government, raising their sense of identity, and making them feel psychologically secure.

In the meantime, China's response to the sources of psychological insecurity associated with covid-19 also fed nationalism and made it thriving during the crisis. As Druckman (1994) insightfully pointed out, although nationalism is conventionally recognised as a political, economic and sociological phenomenon, to a certain extent it is more of a socio-psychological phenomenon manifested in the attitudes that human minds develop towards their own and other nations. At the individual level, nationalism is regarded as one of the psychological consequences to relieve public anxiety resulting from a social environment of uncertainty and fear (Bieber 2020). Accordingly, advancing nationalism in China is not only the very answer to the psychological demands for security in the era of a global pandemic, but also a key to legitimising ideology to sustain power in post-pandemic China. In the combat against covid-19, the most remarkable set of ideologies[13] perceived that aligned with the erewhile emerging covid-related nationalism is the complex of patriotism intertwined with the consciousness of the Chinese nation community. The logic behind this complex of ideologies simply falls on the insistence that the national identity reinvented and solidarity demonstrated amid the pandemic are the reasons for defeating covid-19 in China and they may be even more crucial to the challenges ahead.

In a paper examining whether nationalism emerged globally during the covid-19 pandemic, it is found that the rise of nationalism requires a matching ideology to gain public support (Su and Shen 2021). In the light of this, elevating patriotism and strengthening the sense of the Chinese national community is thus considered more necessary than ever, as it allows for a cost-efficient recovery, growth, and confidence rebuilding from a post-pandemic world by simply responding to the people's demands for (socio-)psychological security, which range from the needs for basic psychological security, to the fulfilment of the supreme ideal of the great rejuvenation of the Chinese national. This clearly explains why, amidst the surge in global nationalist sentiment caused by the public health crisis, China has shown itself to be in an unswerving pursuit of ideologies such as patriotism and the Chinese national community in responding to psychological insecurity of hostility and uncertainty, and in dispelling criticism and negative comments about the government at home and abroad.

[13] It has been described that China has no coherent ideology, what it follows is pragmatism namely anything found workable to deliver growth (Brown 2012).

Cultivating Patriotism: the Party Leadership and Security Agenda in Schools

"Either the Party (CCP itself), politics, military, the Chinese people, and education, or east, west, south, north, and middle, the Party is supposed to lead everything[14]". With this description of the Party's leadership enshrined as a fundamental political principle in its constitution in 2017, the process of democratisation in China has been brought to a complete halt. From then on, CCP's control over ideology, especially over that of in education, has become even heavier. Clearly, the significance of education on shaping young minds and forming a favourable socioeconomic environment for development is very much considered crucial in perpetuating the communist regime. Since 2014, the role of education in fostering moral virtue and people's cultivation has been repeatedly emphasised by President Xi Jinping on various occasions, and there are increasing indications that ideo—moral and political education has become the priority of educational policy agenda in China.

Examples can be drawn from the themes that the Ministry of Education (MOE) sets each Teacher's Day—it is "promoting noble teachers' morality, fostering character and civic virtue (of students)" in 2018 and "strengthening moral education and cultivating responsibility, lifting poverty through education" in 2020—which the themes explicitly reflect the objectives and aspirations of the authority for education. Before the 2020 Teacher's Day, Xi offered a concrete methodology in carrying out his idea on education, by strengthening the role of ideo-moral and ideo-political courses and rituals in the process of educating.[15] The keywords of those officially approved correctness such as patriotism, faith in CCP, and self-confidence in socialism and the political system are notably resounding in setting up the scene for future education works.

For instance, fostering patriotism is reflected in the *Outline for the Implementation of Patriotic Education in the New Era* issued by the CCP

[14] Literal translation of "党政军民学，东西南北中。党是领导一切的。" An interpretation first made by Mao Zedong on the power of the CCP.

[15] An article titled "*Ideopolitical Courses are Pivotal in Implementing the Fundamental Task of Education* 《思政课是落实立德树人根本任务的关键课程》" published by President Xi Jinping in the journal of *QiuShi* 《求是》, one of the most important party newspaper and journal of CCP.

Central Committee and the State Council in 2019, which clearly stipulates the need to make young people the key target of patriotic education. The *Outline* defines patriotism in the Chinese context and specifies the contents of patriotic-related aspects that one shall be organised to learn, including but not limited to educations on the Chinese Dream, national spirit, realities of the country, history of the Party, fine traditional Chinese culture, national reunification (Taiwan), ethnic solidarity, and national security. In other words, educating and learning about any aspect of the aforesaid encompasses the understanding of patriotism in the Chinese context. This shows that patriotism is set to be multidimensional in China, and one must satisfy all the above aspects to be patriotic.

Xi attaches great importance to patriotism and has stressed it many times on different occasion. For example, at the Gathering Marking the Centenary of the May Fourth Movement in April 2019, Xi redefined the patriotism in contemporary China as "upholding a high degree of unity amongst love of the country, the Party and socialism"; and in May 2018 at Peking University Student and Teacher Symposium, Xi elevated patriotism to the premise of a person's "learning to be" by quoting from Sun Yat-sen "the most important thing to be a man is to know how to be patriotic". As the matter of fact, the education for patriotism has never been slackened in China. In most cases, the core of ideopolitical education in China remains essentially the same despite its content and form of delivery may vary in light of different situations at home and abroad. Among them, the education for patriotism seems to be an appropriate solution in responding to students' psychological needs arising from the pandemic.

According to Luo et al. (2020) the underlying issue for the education for patriotism in China today is to generate a sense of national dignity and self-confidence by promoting patriotism. In this sense, battling with the pandemic has given a lot of room for education to play on ideological building over the minds of youth. Due to a strict national lockdown policy, China has been able to contain the spread of the coronavirus in a few months and schools across the country started to resume classes in April. This comes at a time when the coronavirus has just started to plague and cause a surge in confirmed cases and deaths in other affected countries. Although officially China has offered assistance to many of them and organisations as well, the act of giving aid and support itself has tactically become a propaganda element in both online and offline classrooms and has been hailed as the deeds which show "the demeanour of a great nation".

For example, schools have been instructed to carry out patriotic education in response to any covid-related psychological insecurity and ideological dissension that school students may have. The instructions[16] are found both at the national and regional level. At the national level, the MOE had specified the "key content" of carrying out extensive, in-depth and sustained patriotic education among all Party cadres, teachers and students across the country. Among the elements of patriotic education stipulated by the MOE, for instance, are "vividly highlighting the advantages of the socialist system with Chinese characteristics" and "vigorously promoting the spirit of patriotism in the new era". At the local level, based on my empirical research on the patriotic education in Ningxia Hui Autonomous Region (China), where the schools had been instructed to act fast on organising their teachers, Party cadres, supervisors of Young Pioneers and the Communist Youth League for educational propaganda and the forming of patriotism at school. It is worth noting that, according to the document, the education providers and governors at lower levels are required to report on progress to their superiors, which means how well or insufficiently the ideopolitical task of inspiring patriotic enthusiasm is accomplished will be checked and recorded, and as evidence, they will form the basis for future promotions or evaluations.

In short, the CCP's patriotism cultivating effort has long been laying out for the political stability and state security of the party-state. Given the special role of education, schools have always been put in an important place to solidify ideology. Based on the discussion so far, patriotic education is an important part of schools' ideology works even before

[16] There are two circulars from education authorities give an outline of the subsequent patriotic education work and set out the objectives to be achieved at different stages: "Notice on carrying out propagandistic education, collecting and displaying online cultural achievements themed 'Jointly Combating the covid-19 Pandemic and Exercising Patriotism' [关于开展 "共抗疫情、爱国力行"主题宣传教育和网络文化成果征集展示工作的通知] (Ministry of Education Office 2020)", and "Notice on fully exploring educational elements showed during the pandemic and deeply carrying out ideopolitical education works for students [关于充分挖掘抗击疫情中的育人元素深入开展学生思想政治教育工作的通知] (Office of Ningxia Education Working Committee and Education Department 2020)". The two circulars are believed of great political significance to organise schools to fully explore the educational elements of the covid pandemic and carry out ideopolitical education for students in order to protect the *health* of teachers and students, and maintain the *stability* of education institutions.

covid-19, and the pandemic certainly has provided the most seasonable teaching material for patriotic education which in turn justifies the security or liberty of individuals who might be compromised for the sake of "larger picture".

The First Lesson: Dispelling Psychological Insecurity and "Mental Contamination" with Patriotism

During the national lockdown, all teaching and learning were moved online to minimise health risk and the influence on students' academic performance. Meanwhile, screens had become the window for psychological stability and ideological transmission. A side story in *Guangming Daily* in February 2020 reported on a junior high school in Beijing, for example, where students received patriotic education through online classes at home during the outbreak; besides, over 500 students were organised to attend a live streaming flag-raising ceremony on Douyin (Jin et al. 2020) (Figs. 5.1 and 5.2).

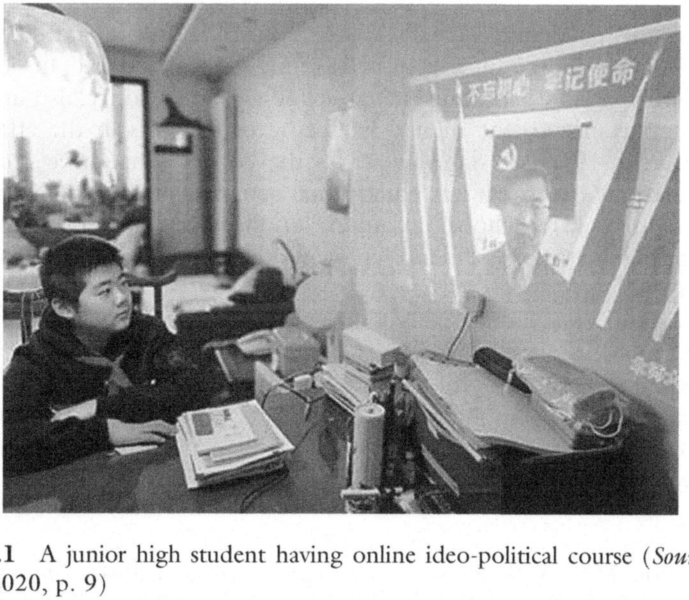

Fig. 5.1 A junior high student having online ideo-political course (*Source* Jin et al. 2020, p. 9)

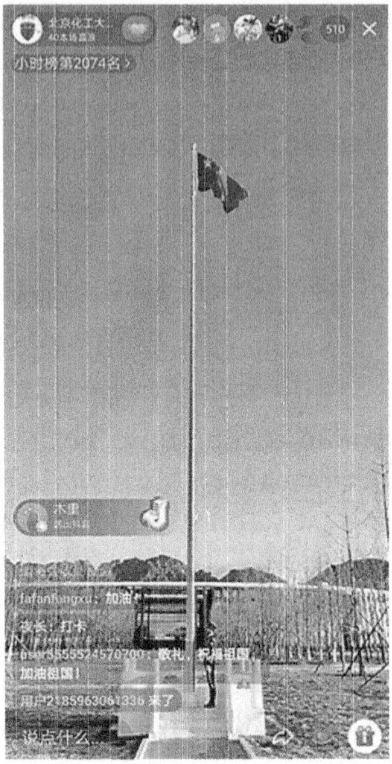

Fig. 5.2 Flag-raising ceremony live streaming on Douyin (*Source* Jin et al. 2020)

With the pandemic virtually under control, primary and secondary schools across the country resumed offline classes in April. In addition to essential covid-19 precautions at schools, the authority also attached great importance to the mental wellbeing of students in the aftermath of the covid-19 crisis. Schools across the country that have reopened were instructed to carry out educational activities on the theme of "the first lesson back to school" in aiming at alleviating any post-lockdown stress or eliminating any "incorrect" views that might occur in classrooms (Fig. 5.3).

According to a Xinhua.net report, on the first day back to school, a junior high school in Haikou city carried out educational activities to strengthen the education for patriotism and enhance the "sense of mission and responsibility" among Grade 9 students (Wang, 2020). By tracing back to this particular school's post on Meipian,[17] more details emerged that were not disclosed by Xinhua.net. For example, the head of school

[17] Meipian 美篇 is a Chinese social media tool for authors and editors to create and beautify images and posts. Many schools in China use Meipian to publicise and keep a

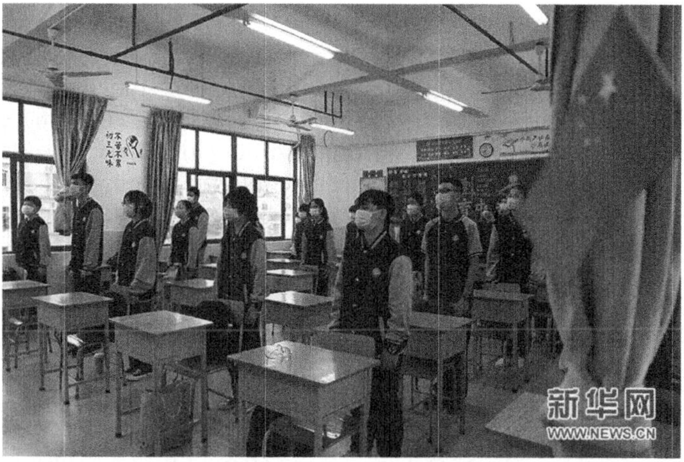

Fig. 5.3 Students perform the flag-raising ceremony in the classroom (*Source* Wang 2020)

Zhang Jian delivered a speech on encouraging students to be patriotic after the indoor flag-raising ceremony by saying:

> ...[this] special term break is also a special educational lesson for all our students. I believe that we who have experienced this are meant to be extraordinary as now we are passionate, and our dreamboat is fully loaded with patriotic and national feelings! I believe our country will emerge stronger from such a pandemic! ... [I hope] you all grow up to be a loving, responsible, professional and contributory adult. (Haikou Yusha Junior High 2020)

This speech was followed by audience students taking a pledge of patriotism. The students are instructed to raise and fist the right hand while repeating after the lead student oath-taker. According to the school's post, the students took the oath of "pride of being Chinese" and swore to be "hardworking for the country's future" and to be "grateful to those who contributed to China's successes". Furthermore, for better effect, the students were kept actively engaged in the topic instead of being imbued

trail of their works, especially the Party, Communist Youth League, and Young Pioneers -related works.

with idea from rituals. More chances were given within classrooms, under the guidance of "class tutors", for peers to share and discuss. In the case of Yusha Junior High, several ideological aspects of students such as the "Three Loves" (refer to "loves of the country, knowledge and work") were projected to be reshaped in combination with China's virus control efforts and results, stories of "advanced people" in fighting against covid-19, and contrasts of the situation in present between China and other countries, on which topics students were expected to share their own opinions and conclude with their reinforced patriotic feelings and strong wills to build the nation (Figs. 5.4 and 5.5).

The above employs Yusha Junior High in Haikou city as the lens to unfold the ideological dynamics of schools across the country when they reopened in April. As part of the new round of the state's educational priorities, patriotic education has been carried out throughout the country against the backdrop of covid-19 with essentially the same outlook and approach as demonstrated at Yusha Junior High.

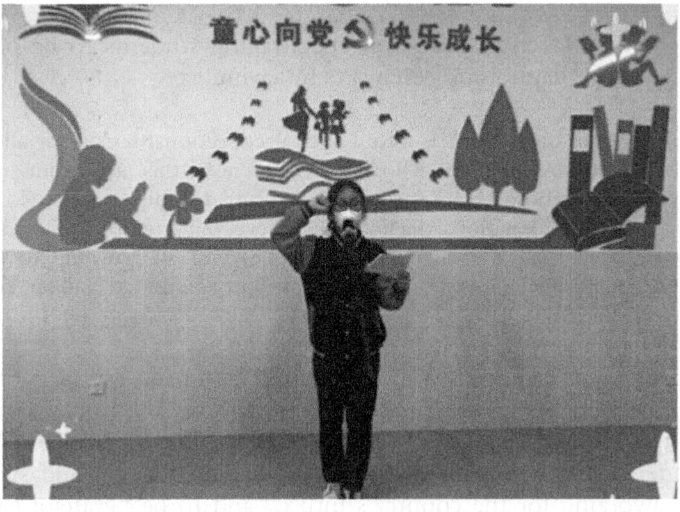

Fig. 5.4 The lead student oath-taker on speaker. The political slogan on the wall behind: "children's hearts are with the Party, and grow up happily" (*Source* Haikou Yusha Junior High 2020)

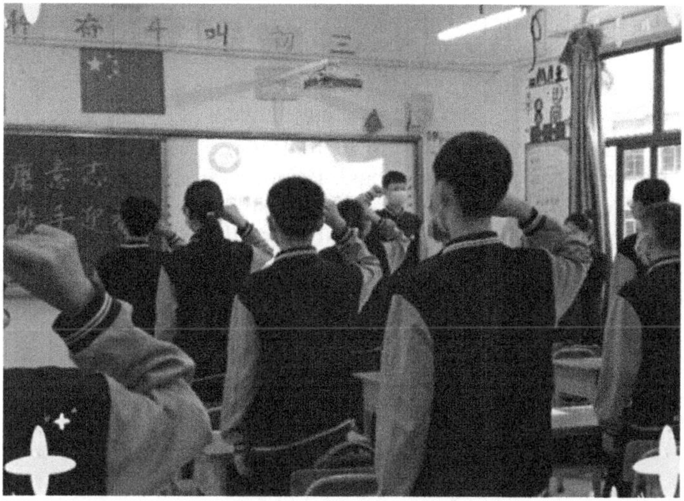

Fig. 5.5 Students of the class all standing still and following the lead of taking an oath (*Source* Haikou Yusha Junior High 2020)

At the national level, a television programme that has been on the air for many years, "*The Frist Class*",[18] has ideologically focussed part of its 2020 episode on combining the covid-19 pandemic with nationalist thinking and ultimately served the growth of patriotism among young Chinese students. The programme begins with a speech delivered by Zhong Nanshan, a Chinese pulmonologist, the leading advisor for covid-19, and the recipient of the highest order of honour Order of the Republic, who first introduced the influence of witnessing the history of the Chinese nation struggling against Japan from the late-1930s to

[18] *The First Class* (《开学第一课》), A television programme jointly produced by the Ministry of Propaganda, the Ministry of Education and China Central Television for primary and secondary school students nationwide. The programme has been broadcast every year since 2008, before the start of the summer term. The programme takes the form of a class meeting session, simulating a classroom, and interacts with students and parents in the audience of the programme by inviting renowned experts, scholars, and social figures. The content of the programme is based on "positive" characters and events, which are used to educate students, especially on patriotism and nationalism. The 2019 episode themed "the Five-Starred Red Flag, I'm proud of you"; and 2020 one themed "the Young is Strong, the Country is Strong".

mid-1940s on his own patriotic beliefs and the ambition to serve China (CCTV-1, 2020, 05:23–07:06), and then endorsed the CCP leadership and governance philosophy displayed during public health crises:

> At that time, the central government took it very seriously after hearing [that the unknown virus is infectious]. President Xi said that the safety and health of our people's lives must be put first, and we must do whatever it takes for that. We would rather shut down the economy than put our people's safety and health at risk. This is very different between us, China, where is under the leadership of the Party, and some countries. First of all, lives matter most. (CCTV, 2020, 11:12–11:49)

Zhong also responded the concerns over human rights that enforced lockdown and movement restrictions are violations:

> [Wuhan], this heroic city, for 76 days and 1,786 hours, [the regional lockdown] was exchanged for allowing China to reduce the number of confirmed cases by at least 700,000. What is this? This is [the principle that] our country sticks to at the soonest, [i.e.] nothing is more precious than lives. What is the greatest human right? It is people's right to life. We have saved the lives of so many people and this is a demonstration of our greatest human right. (12:16–12:50)

It is not difficult to see that part of Zhong's views on some countries' precautions has a nationalistic bent in which his unspoken words left to the understanding of the audience is that China's success in the combat against covid-19 depends to a large extent on institutional strengths, and the organising capacity and decisiveness that China has shown in the process is unparalleled in a democratic system. However, it is clearly lopsided to insinuate that *some countries* lack concern for their peoples' lives by not taking the fact that the decision-making processes and political dilemmas of each country can be disparate into account. Zhong's words ostensibly intended to stir up a feeling of love for and pride in China among the younger generation, are set up in a way that is inconsistent with what China is claiming in its fundamental foreign policy regarding the rational mindset or logic it is based upon. In other words, the cultivation of nationalism in the younger generation of China seems to be slightly different in its mindset from the nationalism that China paraded to the world: in contrast to the latter, the nationalism rhetoric locks China into a Darwinian struggle for survival in which only the strong survive, yet in the diplomatic arena the nationalism that China does not emphasise competition, but rather dialogue, cooperation, and peaceful co-existence.

Patriotism qualifies as a buzzword for this programme. The portrayal of the show's guests, including a student who has been cured of covid-19, and representatives of key workers and Party members who have worked on the front line in Wuhan, generally reflects some of these characteristics: dedication, commitment, solidarity, and self-confidence. For example, Zhang Dingyu, the Head of Wuhan Jinyintan Hospital and Deputy Director of Hubei Provincial Health Commission, who has been suffered from Amyotrophic lateral sclerosis yet still working tirelessly with an unshakable commitment to save lives and said:

> ...suddenly, the phone rang, a medical team of 450 people from the ground force, navy and air force of the People's Liberation Army was about to arrive in Wuhan in 3 hours...this is the strong support that our Party and country sent to my hospital and Wuhan as well. (37:33–39:00)

> ... [those cured Wuhan people,] donated blood plasma with antibodies [to covid-19] which have played a huge role in saving the lives of critically ill patients in other parts of China. We Chinese often say that we are linked by blood. At this moment, we are close to our country. We are never alone in this fight. (41:19–42:00)

Two points are highlighted in Zhang's speech, who first attributed the safety and health of Chinese people in face of covid-19 as a way to inspire gratitude in his young audience and then stressed that the long-lasting collectivist culture of China has been fully vindicated by the crisis. Following his speech and the interview with the host, Zhang's physical condition marked him as a role model who "fights for his beliefs and has achieved self-worth despite being in adversity" in an attempt to indoctrinate the pupils that the younger generation shall be holding the same ideals as lofty as the ones that previous generations have held.

Other guests of role model presented at the show including Mao Qing, healthcare specialist from the army (47:40), Zhang Boli, a specialist in traditional Chinese medicine (58:12), Chen Wei, Chief Researcher of China's covid-19 vaccines (1:04:55), Zhang Wenhong, "ambassador of wearing face-covering" and professor in infectious disease of Tsinghua University (1:09:42), Wu Zunyou, chief epidemiologist of China's Centre for Disease Control (1:15:50), and Xie Jun, Chief Designer of Beidou

Global Navigation Satellite Systems (1:18:50) who demonstrated the country's hard and soft power from the perspectives of the Party and state support, traditional culture, science and technology respectively to stimulate patriotic enthusiasm, solidarity, dedication, self-confidence, and gratitude as well as to form the belief and a sense of mission in serving the country among Chinese students. This TV programme, at the start of a new academic year, is undoubtedly a great inspiration to the audience students like it, in many dimensions, shows the power that distinguishes China from it was a century ago. As will be discussed shortly, all schools from my fieldwork require students to watch *The First Class* in and after class and to talk about it either orally or in writing. Based on the audience's positive feedback that the programme is much admired and held in obligatory regard in schools.

Nevertheless, through this phenomenon of huge popularity and quasi obligation of the students in China, it is important to note the essence behind i.e. the dynamic relationship under the public health crisis between people's need for security (both physical and phycological) and the state's capacity of providing such a source of security. China's covid strategy has proved to be effective in providing sufficient physical protection and security so that students are able to return to school before long. Besides, the Party's response of blowing an ideo-political whirlwind in schools to the animosity, stigma, discrimination, and racism kicked up outside as well as the hesitation, uncertainty, distrust, and dissidence potentially permeated at home and among young minds is thus respectively the countermeasure and initiative for unfavourable political climate both internationally and domestically. Since contrasts between China and other countries on their covid strategies and results are widely used in propaganda, it has to be said that such an ideo-political whirlwind has not only intensified the patriotic and nationalist sentiments amongst the children and youth but has also brought about concerns of chauvinistic trend in China's basic education.

Discussion

As the impact of covid-19 on people's lives deepens, rising nationalism around the world may exacerbate the tensions that already existed between countries. Panic and misrepresentation have made the world landscape more conservative, which is driving deglobalisation. The once prevalent Sinophobic sentiments and discriminatory behaviours in the news reports have sensitised the Chinese nerves.

This chapter illuminates how "psychological security" has been included into the human security agenda of the Chinese state, and how these constructed "security threats" have been tackled through patriotic education in schools. In the face of foreign hostilities, whooping patriotism with nationalist reporting and teaching seems to be the CCP's solution for external hostility, stigma, discrimination, and racism in dispelling the sense of insecurity of Chinese people. Meanwhile, patriotic education also confuses internal hesitation, uncertainty, mistrust, and dissent so that the CCP leadership may continue to favour an irrefutable position. All in all, the handling of the covid outbreak in China has been highly politicised in terms of the necessary psychological interventions that have been found either outside or inside schools.

Earlier in this chapter, the psychological intervention (education for patriotism) in school students has been discussed thoroughly in the context of the Chinese government combating covid-19. However, it seems that it is not only the students who get the most profound patriotic education but also the education professionals. As the front line of propaganda, teachers' commitment to the ideology largely determines whether the "red gene"—the revolutionary spirit that facilitated the founding of the CCP—is passed on without a hitch to the next generation. The sense of insecurity of teachers is supposed to be stronger than that of students who have narrow access to, and lack the ability to interpret, more information. Therefore, holding teachers accountable for the advocacy and not being "mentally contaminated", based on their greater exposure to the insecurity, can instead make teachers themselves more accommodated to patriotic obsession. In this sense, the focus of ideopolitical whirlwinds is on students, but not entirely on them. This logic is crucial to the understanding of the CCP's rationale for appropriating the concept of human security in the Chinese context. In the face of unfavourable international environments, the CCP's approach to human security is inevitably tinted with peculiar "Chinese characteristics" that focus on forging loyalty and maintaining its legitimacy.

References

Bieber, F. 2020. Global Nationalism in Times of the COVID-19 Pandemic. *Nationalities Papers*, pp. 1–13.

Bourdieu, P. and Passeron, J.-C. 1990. *Reproduction in Education, Society and Culture*, 1st ed. London: Sage.

Brown, K. 2012. *The Communist Party of China and Ideology* [Online]. [Accessed 27 April 2021]. Available from: http://muse.jhu.edu/journals/chn/summary/v010/10.2.brown.html.

Brown, P. 2018. *Routledge Revivals: Schooling Ordinary Kids (1987): Inequality, Unemployment, and the New Vocationalism* [Online]. Taylor and Francis. [Accessed 11 May 2021]. Available from: https://www.taylorfrancis.com/books/mono/10.4324/9781351009720/schooling-ordinary-kids-phillip-brown.

Coates, M. 2020. Covid-19 and the Rise of Racism. *The BMJ*. **369**.

Druckman, D. 1994. *Nationalism, Patriotism, and Group Loyalty: A Social Psychological Perspective*.

Global Times 2020. *Some Countries Slow to Respond to Virus*. [Accessed 26 April 2021]. Available from: https://www.globaltimes.cn/content/1180541.shtml.

Guba, E.G. and Lincoln, Y.S. 1994. Competing Paradigms in Qualitative Research In: N.K. Denzin and Y.S. Lincoln, eds. *Handbook of Qualitative Research*. Thousand Oaks, CA; London: SAGE Publications Inc., pp. 105–117.

Haikou Yusha Junior High 2020. "Haikou Yusha Junior High 2020 Spring Grade 9 Students the First Lesson Back to School Educational Activities [海口市玉沙实验学校开展2020年春季初三年级开学典礼暨'疫情磨意志，携手迎春天'开学第一课主题教育]." *Meipian*.

Hatch, J.A. 2002. *Doing Qualitative Research in Education Settings*. Albany: State University of New York Press.

Hswen, Y., Xu, X., Hing, A., Hawkins, J.B., Brownstein, J.S. and Gee, G.C. 2021. Association of "#covid19" Versus "#chinesevirus" with Anti-Asian Sentiments on Twitter: March 9–23, 2020. *American Journal of Public Health*. **111**(5), pp. 956–964.

Huanqiu Shibao 2020. "Editorial: We Are Concerned That Some Countries Are a Bit Slow to Act on Prevention and Control [社评: 我们担心，一些国家防控行动有点慢]." *Global Times Editorial Collection* [Online]. [Accessed 26 April 2021]. Available from: https://opinion.huanqiu.com/article/9CaKrnKpxZm.

Jin, X., Yao, Xi. and Tang, Q. 2020. "First Class Online: The Covid as Textbook 线上开学第一课: 把疫情当教科书." *Guangming Daily* [Online], p. 9. [Accessed 6 May 2021]. Available from: https://epaper.gmw.cn/gmrb/html/2020-02/18/nw.D110000gmrb_20200218_1-09.htm.

Lee, R.K.-W. and Li, Z. 2021. Online Xenophobic Behavior Amid the COVID-19 Pandemic. *Digital Government: Research and Practice*. **2**(1), pp. 1–5.

Lemke, T. 2011. *Biopolitics: An Advanced Introduction* [Online]. New York and London: NYU Press. [Accessed 16 April 2021]. Available from: https://www.jstor.org/stable/j.ctt9qg0rd.

Li, Y. and Nicholson, H.L. 2021. When "Model Minorities" Become "Yellow Peril"—Othering and the Racialization of Asian Americans in the COVID-19 Pandemic. *Sociology Compass*. **15**(2).

Luo, W., Ding, Y. and Kuang, X. 2020. Chinese Students' Attitudes Toward Patriotism Education. In: K.J. Kennedy, ed. *Social Studies Education in East Asian Contexts*. Oxon and New York: Routledge, pp. 125–135.

Ministry of Education Office 2020. "Notice on Carrying Out Propagandistic Education, Collecting and Displaying Online Cultural Achievements Themed 'Jointly Combating the covid-19 Pandemic and Exercising Patriotism' [关于开展'共抗疫情、爱国力行'主题宣传教育和网络文化成果征集展示工作的通知]."

Misra, S., Le, P.T.D., Goldmann, E. and Yang, L.H. 2020. Psychological Impact of Anti-Asian Stigma Due to the COVID-19 Pandemic: A Call for Research, Practice, and Policy Responses. *Psychological Trauma: Theory, Research, Practice, and Policy*. **12**(5), p. 461.

Office of Ningxia Education Working Committee and Education Department 2020. "Notice on Fully Exploring Educational Elements Showed During the Pandemic and Deeply Carrying Out Ideopolitical Education Works for Students [关于充分挖掘抗击疫情中的育人元素深入开展学生思想政治教育工作的通知]" [Online]. Available from: http://jyt.nx.gov.cn/sviewp/AF04663A-6196-406A-85DD-75A54D29DDA8.

Parsons, T. 2008. The School Class as a Social System In: J.H. Ballantine and J.Z. Spade, eds. *Schools and Society: A Sociological Approach to Education*. London: Pine Forge Press, pp. 80–85.

Saltman, K.J. 2018. *The Politics of Education: A Critical Introduction*, 2nd ed. New York and Oxon: Routledge.

Sen, A. 2002. *Basic Education and Human Security* [Online]. Kolkata. [Accessed 16 April 2021]. Available from: https://afed.itacec.org/document/Education%20and%20Human%20Security.pdf.

Shavit, Y. and Müller, W. 2006. Vocational Secondary Education, Tracking, and Social Stratification In: *Handbook of the Sociology of Education* [Online]. Springer US, pp. 437–452. [Accessed 17 April 2021]. Available from: https://link.springer.com/chapter/10.1007/0-387-36424-2_20.

Su, R. and Shen, W. 2021. Is Nationalism Rising in Times of the COVID-19 Pandemic? Individual-Level Evidence from the United States. *Journal of Chinese Political Science*. **26**(1), pp. 169–187.

Tahmasbi, F., Schild, L., Ling, C., Blackburn, J., Stringhini, G., Zhang, Y. and Zannettou, S. 2021. "Go Eat a Bat, Chang!": On the Emergence of Sinophobic Behavior on Web Communities in the Face of COVID-19. *Proceedings of the Web Conference 2021, Association for Computing Machinery* (pp. 1122–1133). New York, NY, USA. Available from: https://doi.org/10.1145/3442381.3450024.

UNDP. 1994. *Human Development Report*. New York and Oxford.
Wang, W. 2020. "The First Class Back to School 疫情后的开学第一课." *Xinhua.net* [Online]. [Accessed 6 May 2021]. Available from: http://m.xinhuanet.com/hq/2020-04/07/c_1125821614.htm.
Zhao, L. 2020. 2/2 美国疾控中心主任被抓了个现行。零号病人是什么时候在美国出现的?有多少人被感染?医院的名字是什么?可能是美军把疫情带到了武汉。美国要透明!要公开数据!美国欠我们一个解释! [Twitter]. [Accessed 11 May 2021]. Available from: https://twitter.com/zlj517/status/1238113459234934785?s=20.

CHAPTER 6

Immobility: Surviving the COVID-19 Outbreak

Qiyang Liu

Introduction

"A new concept of human security" that shifts the focus from conflicts between nations to deliverable security for individuals within nations in their daily lives was first proposed in the United Nations Development Program (UNDP)'s *Human Development Report 1994* (UNDP 1994). This concept focuses on emerging concerns of individuals which were previously less pertained within the security discourse, such as job security, income security, health security, environmental security and security from crime. The concept of people-centred human security was further elaborated by the report of the independent Commission on Human Security *Human Security Now* (CHS 2003), stating that "(human security) requires both shielding people from acute threats and empowering people to take charge of their own lives" and therefore Governments should implement "integrated policies that focus on people's survival,

Q. Liu (✉)
School of Urban Planning and Design, Peking University Shenzhen Graduate School, Shenzhen, China
e-mail: tsql@pku.edu.cn

C. Zhang (ed.), *Human Security in China*,
https://doi.org/10.1007/978-981-16-4675-1_6

livelihood, and dignity during downturns as well as in prosperity". Human security, albeit ambiguous in its conceptualisation and overlapping implications with social exclusion which has been increasingly a focus in the transport domain (see Lucas 2012, 2019), offers a new approach to rethink transport-related social issues that may be underexplored within the existing transport and human security literatures.

"The number of years of future life spent outside a state of 'generalised poverty'" (King and Murray 2001) was used as the definition of human security throughout this chapter. Under this definition, several components of human security have been discussed in the transport literature, including (a) transport poverty (see Lucas et al. 2016 for a review), which focuses on exploring the cause-of and caused-by relations between transport and poverty, such as transport affordability (e.g., Litman 2015), fuel poverty (e.g., Walker and Day 2012), mobility poverty (e.g., Salon and Gulyani 2010), accessibility poverty (e.g., Velaga et al. 2012), and exposure to transport externalities (e.g., Barter 1999); (b) transport disadvantage, which concerns transport-related social disadvantages, such as the outcome of a lack of access to essential resources, activities and opportunities (e.g., Schwanen et al. 2015); (c) accessibility, which has been the centre of academic attention for researchers in the field of both transport and planning since 1970s (Handy 2020), concerning the ease with which activities can be reached (see Geurs and van Wee 2004 for a review) and (d) transport-related social exclusion (see Lucas 2006, 2012, 2019; Liu et al. 2019), which systematically examines how people may be socially excluded by the transport system, in the following seven aspects: physical, geographical, economic, time-based, fear-based, space exclusion and exclusion from facilities (Church et al. 2000). These theoretical and empirical efforts have elucidated how the transport system may contribute to a state of generalised poverty, although they were not intended to make a connection with the concept of human security.

The ongoing COVID-19 pandemic, which struck 192 countries and territories, causing more than 2.28 million deaths by the end of January 2021, is the defining global health crisis of our time. Due to this greatest challenge humanity faced since World War Two, nations' governance and societal responses have been put to the test. Governments have implemented various policy interventions to contain the outbreak of COVID-19 in both the Global North and South, such as quarantine, social distancing, curfew laws, school closure, gathering restrictions and lockdown measures. Despite the widely extolled containing effects of these measures (e.g., Gatto et al. 2020), their social consequences are still underexplored. This pandemic has surfaced concerns which has been practically unnoticeable and much less talked about in the transport domain, for example, the ease of acquiring preferred food, the important role of social interactions while walking and how travel and outdoor activities might be influenced by cyberbullying and real-life bullying.

To fill this void, this chapter aims to examine the (im)mobility of lay-citizens during the COVID-19 pandemic by employing the human security approach. In so doing, this study contributes to the literature in three aspects: (a) identifying two distinct groups of people during the pandemic—the imposed immobility and the self-motivated immobility group; (b) understanding attitudes and needs of the imposed immobility group who have been in a state of insecurity throughout the pandemic; (c) discussing issues that have not been considered as potentially connected to the transport system, such as food security.

Methodology

This study involves the collection and analysis of two dataset. Qualitative data, collected from interview, was first used to explore how and why people respond to COVID-19 and its corresponding policies and then a monthly panel survey was used to investigate the impact of COVID-19 containment measures and attitudinal and behavioural change during work resumption. The qualitative exploration is needed to understand the complex nature of the social impacts of COVID-19 and inform the questionnaire design. Then quantitative data, collected from a survey is needed to collect measurable behaviour and attitudes and verify findings from the qualitative study.

The Studied Case

The study took place in the city of Kunming in Southwest China. Kunming was selected as the case for this study for three main reasons.

(a) Kunming, as the third biggest city in Southwest China, shares similar economic, social and spatial characteristics with other large Chinese cities. As of 2019, Kunming had a total population of 6.95 million and an urban population of 5.11 million (Bureau of Statistics of Kunming 2020).

(b) Kunming is a representative case in terms of the seriousness of COVID-19 and containment interventions. COVID-19 struck Yunnan at the end of January, with 187 reported confirmed cases, including two deaths to date. In the early phase of the outbreak, the Government discouraged residents from participating in social activities; applied closed-off management to residential areas; shut down public transport; closed business zones, parks, schools and universities and forbade rural residents from travelling to the city. Since late February, a precision containment strategy was adopted in response to the call for work resumption. The strategy involved a risk-based regulation, which lifted travel restrictions on residents in low-risk regions (see Xinhua News 2020) and implemented a smartphone-based health-tracking system (see Mozur et al. 2020). The situation is similar to most other Chinese cities, except for cities in Hubei Province and other centres of the outbreak, such as Wenzhou.

(c) Yunnan province was one of the six provinces that reported no confirmed cases of SARS infection. Yunnan and Tibet were the only two provinces that have never shrouded in fear about SARS, as no suspected cases had arisen during the SARS pandemic (Ministry of Health 2003). Residents in Kunming were anticipated to concern less about the novel coronavirus than those who had experienced similar situations during the SARS pandemic in the early phase of the pandemic. Therefore, it would be easier to observe behavioural and attitudinal changes during the pandemic.

Data Collection and Analysis

Several different approaches were adopted to reach diverse people because Chinese people are generally unwilling to talk about inner feelings and actual opinions with strangers, especially when face-to-face conversations were perceived dangerous. These approaches include (detailed recruiting process see Liu et al. 2021b): (a) making the acquaintance of older people by walking and staying in the residential areas where they lived and talking with them informally; (b) inviting participants recruited by the first approach to introduce their acquaintances living in other residential areas; (c) snow-ball sampling; recruiting in public spaces after the lifting of restrictions.

Table 6.1 Information about the interviewees

		Number	*Proportion/%*
Gender	Male	227	43.7
	Female	292	56.3
Age	≥65	248	47.8
	40–64	161	31.0
	≤ 39	110	21.2
Household size	1	21	4.0
	2	130	25.0
	3	192	37.0
	4	103	19.8
	>4	73	14.1

A total of 186 families with 519 residents participated in family interviews. Among them, 248 were older than 65, 161 participants were aged between 40 and 64 and 110 participants were younger than 40. Information about the interviewees is presented in Table 6.1.

Each family interview lasted average 55 mins, ranging from 41 to 89 mins. Short individual interview with the absent family member lasted average 17 mins, ranging from 7 to 23 mins. Individual interview with family members separately lasted average 24 mins, ranging from 11 to 36 mins. All interviews were recorded and transcribed. All the transcripts were translated into English by the researcher in preparation for subsequent analysis. An inductive category development approach was adopted (Thomas 2006) and the software package NVivo 11 was used to organise, code, categorise and visualise the data. Two rounds of coding were completed independently by Liu and Liu. In order to minimise the extent to which the meaning of content was changed through translation, the Chinese version of transcripts were used in the first round of coding and the translated version were used in the second round. Themes were discussed between co-authors and experts from various fields. A list of 1896 codes ("nodes" in NVivo) were generated, and then categorised into 58 themes ("parent nodes" in NVivo). Several rounds of analyses were carried out after initial coding, including linking themes, selecting representative quotations and theory generation grounded in the data.

In this chapter, quantitative data was only used to identify the imposed and self-motivated immobility groups. Detailed analysis of how disadvantaged people were excluded and marginalised by containment policies and the contemporary practice of smartphone-based new mobility services were discussed in a previous paper (Liu et al. 2021a). Quantitative data used in this study was collected monthly from February to October 2020 in Kunming, China. The participants of family interviews were invited to take and disseminate the survey. 401 of 519 interviewees responded to the survey in the first wave collection. The first wave of data collection took place on February 24–28 with a total of 1572 respondents. All the participants of the first wave data collection were contacted for subsequent surveys but only 569 residents completed all waves of data collection. The socio-demographic characteristics of these respondents are presented in Table 6.2.

K-means clustering was adopted to classify the 569 respondents of the monthly survey based on the characteristics of their travel and outdoor activities during the pandemic. Four variables were used for the clustering: days of outdoor activities per week and self-reported daily travel distance in February, June, and October. The Silhouettes method (Rousseeuw 1987) indicated a three-cluster solution as the optimal number for the cluster analysis. The clustering results are shown in Table 6.3.

Table 6.2 Socio-demographic characteristics of the sample

		Frequency	*Percentage*
Age	18–30	87	15.3
	31–45	181	31.8
	46–60	143	25.1
	Above 60	158	27.8
Gender	Male	276	48.5
	Female	293	51.5
Monthly household disposable income (CNY)	<6000	167	29.3
	6000–9999	171	30.0
	10,000–19,999	166	29.2
	> 20,000	65	11.4
Employment status	Employed	357	62.7
	Unemployed	52	9.1
	Retired	160	28.1
Residential Area	Within 1st ring road	128	22.5
	Between 1st and 2nd ring road	194	34.1
	Between 2nd and 3rd ring road	183	32.2
	Outside 3rd ring road	64	11.2
Car ownership	Car Owner	249	43.8
	Non-car owner	320	56.2

Table 6.3 Travel behaviours of each segment

	Type I (20%)	*Type II (69%)*	*Type III (11%)*
Feb days of outdoor activities per week	5.77	1.32	0.81
Feb self-reported daily travel distance (km)	2.27	0.35	0.14
Jun days of outdoor activities per week	5.16	5.80	1.33
Jun self-reported daily travel distance (km)	2.93	8.58	0.19
Oct days of outdoor activities per week	5.81	5.86	1.20
Oct self-reported daily travel distance (km)	6.68	8.39	0.18

Imposed and Self-Motivated Immobility

As shown in Table 6.3, the surveyed population fell into three distinct groups with respect to their travel and outdoor behaviours during the pandemic—people in segment I routinely travelled and performed outdoor activities near their residential area in the early phase of the pandemic but the frequency of their outdoor activities and travel distances remained largely unchanged three months after the work resumption; those in segment II had been notably immobile in the early phase of COVID-19 but effectively restored their mobility after the pandemic has been successfully contained; segment III consist of people who mostly stayed at home during the pandemic.

Both type I and type III (immobile) people can be regarded as the imposed immobility group because they cannot restore their mobility when they want to. Although type I people frequently went outside even in the hardest time, their travel distance barely increased three months after the lifting of many travel restrictions. However, their travel distance doubled after the lifting of compulsory QR-code-for-buses which indicated that their travel demand was substantially unmet until the health QR code did not require for taking buses. Therefore, they were still largely immobile because of imposed policy interventions. Type III people were immobile throughout the period of observation. They rarely went out and most trips were within or around the community.

Type II can be regarded as the self-motivated immobility group because they stayed at home in the initial stage of the pandemic and travelled much longer distances and more frequently thereafter. In fact, their travel behaviours remained relatively stable since March (average 5.03 days of outdoor activities per weeks, average 7.35 km self-reported daily travel distance). These results imply that this population group were capable of being mobile even if they were constrained by policy interventions of various sorts. It is therefore evident that for this group, staying immobile in the first few weeks of the pandemic was more of a preference or self-motivated choice depending on the risk of infection and other considerations.

Traditionally in transport studies, travel behaviours have been considered correlated with socio-demographic characteristics. As aforementioned, disadvantaged people are anticipated more likely to suffer from the negative impacts of containment measures during the pandemic. Therefore, investigating the socio-demographic composition of the three segments can deepen our understanding of immobility during the pandemic. As shown in Table 6.4, the imposed immobility groups (types I & III) comprise mostly retired old members while the majority of people in the self-motivated immobility group (type II) are younger working people. Type I people tend to be generally poorer and some three quarters of type I members were in the poorest quartile while type III people

Table 6.4 Social-demographic characteristics of each segment

		Type I (%)	*Type II (%)*	*Type III (%)*
Age	18–30	3.5	19.7	9.2
	31–45	2.7	45.3	1.5
	46–60	15.0	31.5	4.6
	Above 60	78.8	3.6	84.6
Gender	Male	61.1	47.3	33.8
	Female	38.9	52.7	66.2
Monthly household disposable income (CNY)	<6000	73.5	19.9	9.2
	6000–9999	20.3	35.3	15.4
	10,000–19,999	6.2	35.8	29.2
	>20,000	0.0	9.0	46.2
Employment status	Employed	1.8	90.0	4.6
	Unemployed	11.5	8.2	10.8
	Retired	86.7	1.8	84.6

were much richer—around half of its members fall into the richest quartile. This result is implausible because most of the retired cadres who can obtain much more welfare benefits from the level-based cadre retirement treatment (see Manion 2014; Yang et al. 2015) fall into type I, as well as those who are still doing part-time works after retirement. Since only 3 out of 65 type III people are employed, the results suggest that all the elderly people in this group lived with family members in relatively high social positions.

Besides, as presented in Liu et al. (2021a, b), the imposed immobility populations are less technology-savvy, less familiar with smartphone-based services, such as online shopping, banking, social media and new mobility services. Their accessibility to daily necessities and public services highly depends on containment policies, especially the health QR-code-for-buses. Their attitudes towards containment measures had been substantially more negative compared to others predominantly because of their insecure access to food and social interactions.

In short, the imposed immobility group and the self-motivated immobility group have been influenced by COVID-19 differently. The results show a significant shift in mobility behaviour within the self-motivated immobility group—from absolute immobility during the self-perceived "dangerous days" to a high level of mobility after the work resumption; while the imposed immobility group had to remain mobile within the community when their better-off counterparts stayed at home but could not effectively restore mobility as others did.

Insecure Mobility

Six main themes emerged from the qualitative data as mobility-related elements that contribute to a state of "generalised poverty" during the pandemic: insecure access to food, insecure access to facemasks, insecure access to social activities, insecure access to social interactions, a lack of updated information about containment measures and risk of infection due to outdoor activities.

Insecure Access to Food and Other Necessities

The imposed immobility group had experienced varied degrees of difficulties in acquiring daily necessities, especially food and facemasks. Grocery shopping in the first few weeks was the most frequently mentioned issue in family interviews (2033 times in total). The majority of people in the imposed immobility group were used to acquire food from wet markets, most of which were far away from their homes. Since more than three quarters of people from type I were older than 60 who owned public transport courtesy card, they usually took buses and sometimes subways to buy food from wet markets in which they can find their acquaintance shoppers. Most of them would travel longer distances for some particular types of food such as seafood, wild mushroom and wild lives.

However, they can no longer visit these wet markets in the first two to three weeks of the outbreak, not only because the closed-off management was widely applied to residential areas, especially gated community but also because wet markets were closed as they were condemned the scourge of COVID-19. Type I people therefore had to shift to community grocery shops and convenient stores for food acquisition while type II people stayed at home using various online services to acquire food. Compared to the imposed immobility group, self-motivated immobility people had multiple ways to without conducting shopping trips.

Fresh food E-commerce such as *Hemaxiansheng* and *Dingdongmaicai*, offered younger people who had formed the habit of online shopping to easily acquire high-quality food. Although it is not as convenient as usual since they needed to order the food at midnight and take the food at the gate of the community in the first two to three weeks of the pandemic, interviewees from the self-motivated immobility group rarely complained about the difficulties in acquiring food and the quality of food. High-quality fresh (albeit expensive) food was delivered to the gate of their community where people could collect food with a few minutes' walk. To avoid close contact with other people, some type II people paid the gate-keeper of their community to carry the food to the entrance of their flat. Besides, type II people also used social media for food acquisition. For example, many middle-aged people mentioned they had the experience of ordering food from WeChat groups created by community grocers in the early phase of the pandemic. They were regular customers of local grocery shops before the pandemic and had built upon years of relationship between local grocers. Fresh and relatively higher quality food were reserved and directly delivered to their home in the darkest days.

The imposed immobility group, however, had no other ways. Walking to community groceries was the only option. Due to widely reported food safety issues in China (e.g., Lam et al. 2013; Xue and Zhang 2013) and the enduring enthusiasm for life nurturing (e.g., Farquhar and

Zhang 2012), most of the imposed immobility interviewees found food from community groceries extremely intolerable. They "would never buy food from community groceries and convenient stores in normal days" because vegetables in those stores were repeatedly described as expensive, not fresh, low-quality, pesticide and/or preservative overused. Meat in these stores was considered from animals with diseases, ractopamine, and synthetic auxins and consequently less trustworthy. Most of the older and middle-aged interviewees preferred live poultry and livestock raised by farmers who sell such products in wet markets. Although live poultry markets have been identified a major source of various influenzas (e.g., Gilbert et al. 2014), the risk of influenza infection was perceived as accidental compared to the long-lasting risk of "toxic food" from unfamiliar grocery shops. Lacking access to wet markets not only restrained the imposed immobility group from acquiring food they wanted but brought about distrust and anxiety towards their food, and thereby feelings of insecurity during the pandemic.

> *I worried about our food. I haven't eaten any meat for a while, … I don't dare eating meat from those shops. … just one glimpse I know they are meat of dead cows and pigs, pigs died from disease. … The colour of the meat is different; you should never trust those peddlers.* [Female, 77 years old, living with her husband]

Although many interviewees complained that they had to walk an unacceptable distance to acquire food, they started buying food from familiar wet markets right after the lifting of travel restrictions. They acknowledged that long-distance walking might still be dangerous but were willing to take the risks due to the price and perceived safety issue of food from community grocery shops. Their long distance for grocery shopping is mainly a repercussion of a series of urban regeneration projects in Kunming since late 1990s, by which most wet markets around residential areas have been demolished and urban villages where grocery shoppers lived have been erased (see cases from other Chinese cities Wu et al. 2013; Yang and Chang 2007; Zhong and Chen 2017). As one of the interviewees explained:

> *We need more than 50 minutes to walk from home to the nearest wet market. … The market we used some twenty years ago was demolished because of some urban renewal. The government, those corrupt cadres cheated us, saying that*

> *they would build a fancy new one around here but never. We people live in this communityhave been travelling such a long distance for food for more than 20 years! ... It was not a big problem before ... but now this is a very serious problem for us.* [Female, 75 years old, living with her husband]

Because of the high frequency of outdoor activities and facemask shortage, the imposed immobility group had insufficient access to facemasks compared to others in the first two weeks of pandemic (see also Wu et al. 2020). More than half of the imposed immobility people did not wear facemasks when walking and doing grocery shopping in their community. About 40% of them reused disposable facemasks, some even repeatedly used one single facemask for more than one week. Their facemask using behaviour further placed them in a state of insecurity, especially when they were increasingly aware of the severity of the pandemic and risks of outdoor activities without facemasks—although none of them was infected, they had been suffering from perturbation of infection because of lacking facemasks.

In summary, interviewees in the imposed immobility group had remained a state of insecurity in terms of accessibility to acceptable food, suspiciousness of the quality of food, and going out without facemasks. They had experienced household food insecurity because of the community closed-off management in the early phase of the pandemic and compulsory QR-for-buses after the work resumption took place. More importantly, they had been distressed due to their perceptions of community grocers and facemask using.

Insecure Access to Social Interactions and Social Activities

According to King and Murray (2001), "generalised poverty occurs when an individual falls below the threshold of any key domain of human well-being". Social interactions, social activities and social participation have been identified as key dominants of psychological and social well-being (e.g., Cicognani et al. 2008; Huxhold et al. 2014; Ishii-Kuntz 1990; Sharifian and Grühn 2019).

Most of the imposed immobility interviewees lacked the opportunities to interact with others due to containment interventions. Unlike the self-motivated immobility group who can interact with their acquaintances via smartphone-based social media apps, as well as strangers via forum discussion apps, members in the imposed immobility group highly depended on face-to-face interactions. Interestingly, online and mobile games, short-video apps, online shopping apps also offered ways of social interaction for many interviewees under 35 during the pandemic. For these people, the first two weeks of the pandemic was the best of times. As one interviewee explained:

> *I found paradise in those days, staying at home without my mom's nagging. I don't need to work, just laying down. That was awesome. I played Animal Crossing every day with three cyber-friends. We won't have much time to play if there is no COVID-19. ... We chatted with each other all the time, it's hard to feel lonely. It's like living a different life and it was so real when you have nothing else to do. ... I don't even want to go back to normal days.* [Female, 24 years old, living with her parents]

Online and mobile gaming appeared an extremely important form of social activity in the initial stage of the coronavirus pandemic. Online video game play was usually deemed problematic and discouraged by young people's parents because of anticipated negative real-world consequences such as decreasing academic performance, hindering self-esteem, influencing offline relationships with others (e.g., Domahidiet al. 2018; Krossbakken et al. 2018; Toker and Baturay 2016). Since staying at home was preferred in the early stage of the pandemic, offline social activities were hardly accessible. Online gaming therefore offered young people an opportunity for virtual participation in social activities such as organising guild activities, partying, raiding, doing quest with friends and sometimes travelling and taking photos in a virtual world. A noticeable increase in the number of online gamers within young interviewees and the duration of online gaming can be observed. Some of those who had never played video games previously also got into online or mobile games while staying at home. Only two of the online gamers within the young people group felt depressed or lonely in the early phase of the pandemic while more than forty young people reported such mental health issues.

However, older people rarely played any video games and most of the places for social activities where imposed immobility people usually visited were closed or deemed dangerous otherwise, such as green spaces, public parks, outdoor gymnastic apparatuses, card/chess rooms, and tea rooms. Therefore, they can only interact with non-family members during walking. As our previous paper (Liu et al. 2021a) revealed, most of the trips undertaken by imposed immobility people were not for shopping or visiting public services but for fulfilling their social needs. They met, greeted and sometimes chatted with other people when they were walking. According to many imposed immobility interviewees, meeting their acquaintances while walking was already a great relief. Although walking outdoors was perceived somewhat risky, those who regularly walked and met acquaintances outdoors had apparently higher level of mental wellbeing than those who were strongly discouraged from going out. For example, an elderly woman who stayed at home in the first one month of COVID-19 was seriously depressed:

> *I heard from my housemaid, Zeng Hong (an old man living in the same building) had stayed in the hospital for more than one month. I'm pretty sure he got the virus. He always leaves the hospital after two to three weeks but one month this time. He can't make it. … I feel very sick as well, I want to go to the hospital but they (her sons) asked me to wait. I think I got the virus too. There is not much time left for me.* [Female, 92 years old, widowed, living with a housemaid]

Such mental health issue was pervasively found within the very old group (85+). They usually travelled much less frequently than others but these weekly or semi-weekly outdoor activities ensured their connectivity with others. Due to the pandemic, they could not maintain social relationships without regular within-community activities and therefore influenced their psychological and emotional wellbeing (see also Kelly et al. 2017; Nyqvist et al. 2013).

In short, the imposed immobility group had been in a state of insecurity in terms of psychological and social wellbeing because they could not reap the benefits from smartphone-based services. Their social interactions highly depend on face-to-face conversations and their social activities had to be participated outside the home. This partially explained why type I people travelled much more frequently than self-motivated immobility people in the early phase of the pandemic.

As can be seen from the self-reported travel behaviour and concerns about acquiring daily necessities and maintaining social life, the imposed immobility group had to consider the trade-off between the risk of infection and other needs that were perceived more essential to their wellbeing such as food and social interactions. In such circumstances, they often took the risk of COVID-19 infection and kept mobile at least within community. Even so, they had been in a state of insecurity in the early phase of COVID-19 because of lacking access to food they wanted and access to social interactions and social activities.

Physical Abuse and Cyberbullying in the Name of Security

The imposed immobility group had experienced other people's physical abuse during the work resumption and cyberbullying throughout the pandemic in the name of both individual and national security. Consequently, they were unable to restore their mobility which is essential to their wellbeing and therefore in a state of insecurity.

After the work resumption started to take place since the end of February, the Government has implemented a precision containment strategy which lifted the travel restrictions for residents of the community with no confirmed case, gradually reopened business zones, parks, schools and universities, and gradually reopened public transport. For the self-motivated immobility group, a significant escalation of both travel frequency and distance occurred after the lifting of travel restrictions (see Table 6.3). However, as presented in our previous study (Liu et al. 2021a, b), the perceived accessibility to daily necessities and public services of the elderly and low-income people, who compound the type I imposed immobility group, remained at a very low level three months after the lifting of travel restrictions. They could not restore their mobility until the health QR code was no longer compulsory for talking buses. It is because their long-distance travel relies on public transport. Since most of the imposed immobility people were inexperienced smartphone users, they had been intimidated of taking buses because of being incapable of scanning the health QR code and humiliated by other passengers.

Unfriendly attitudes towards and behaviours against elderly people emerged during the pandemic. Many older interviewees were rebuked and humiliated by younger people when they attempted to take buses after the reopening of some bus lines. For example:

> *That day, I wanted to take a bus then the driver asked me to scan the [QR] code. My mobile phone is that kind of phone especially for elderly people ... not a smartphone; it can't do that scanning or maybe I don't know how to use it to scan ... I told the driver, he asked me to get out. I thought that's unfair, so I argued with the driver. Then suddenly those passengers shouted at me*

> *and drove me out.... They said something extremely insulting, like "we don't mind you screw up yourself but don't harm others".... Although there are buses running outside now, we (elderly) are not allowed to use them.* [Male, 77 years old, living with his wife]

About thirty interviewees reported similar experiences of elderly abuse which considerably discouraged their public transport use after the service lockdown was lifted. Many elderly people were afraid of taking buses, not only because of the risk of infection but anticipated hostility from the younger ones. Many elderly people thought this reflected moral degradation of Chinese youth under the influence of Western culture. Younger generations, especially the Generation Z, were perceived as individualists who no longer conform to the cultural norm of respecting the aged. A few older interviewees assumed the hostile behaviours towards the elderly during COVID-19 had emerged from younger public transport users' dissatisfaction with courtesy card holders for their immoderate use of public transport. This can be corroborated by young interviewees who complained about elder bus users. They considered most of the public transport trips undertaken by the elderly unnecessary. As one of the young interviewees explained, "elderly people use public transport for everything because it is free. Actually, they don't have to travel miles for grocery shopping or playing cards". Therefore, these young people thought the elderly should not choose such a high-risk mode for seemingly unnecessary travel during COVID-19. Also, many young people thought older people were extremely uncooperative when boarding the bus, for example many elderly people refused to scan the health QR code and some did not wear facemasks properly. These were naturally connected to widespread reports of shameful behaviours by the elderly (see Wei 2014). Most of the interviewees in the self-motivated immobility group, especially the youth, thought elderly people should stay at home for sake of their own security and others' when younger people themselves started travelling normally. It is evident that these young interviewees denied elderly people's rights to be mobile and hindered them from getting rid of poverty in the name of security.

In the initial stage of COVID-19, staying at home was claimed by many self-motivated immobility people as a patriotic behaviour. For example, "staying at home helps the Government to fight COVID-19", "walking out messes up the country", "everyone should stop making trouble and stay at home", "staying inside home keeps the coronavirus outside home", "we contribute to the society by staying at home". Under this social norm, type I people's routine outdoor activities were accused in spite of the fact that they had to walk out for necessities and social needs. They had been the target of online invectives which extensively reproached them for their "ignorance", "irrationality", "selfishness", "lack of patriotism", "indifference to the pandemic" and "trouble making". Although cyberbullying against those who did not stay at home may not have a direct impact on the targeted people, cyberbullying was found an extension of real-life bullying and those who act as cyberbullies are usually those who bully others in real life (Landstedt and Persson 2014; Riebel et al. 2009). Most of the type I interviewees bore intensive social pressure from others for their only way to acquire daily necessities and participate in social activities.

Interestingly, the self-motivated immobility group promptly restored their mobility after the lifting of some travel restrictions and walking out was suddenly not a troublemaking behaviour anymore. However, after days of blame for walking and outdoor activities, many imposed immobility people stated that they were "afraid of messing up the country if they walked outside the community" after the work resumption took place. Some already lost their motivation to interact with other people because younger family members did not allow them to communicate with others while walking in the early phase of the pandemic. For example:

> *My granddaughter said I can go out only if I guarantee I won't talk to anyone while walking. She said "stop meeting each other so that we can meet each other in the future".... Now, I don't know what to talk about even if I meet those old friends. I can only stand there watching them having a warm chat but I don't know what to say.... I also walk every day alone, that's a bit boring.* [Male, 79 years old, living with his wife]

As the results shown, security has been utilised in the blaming game on the imposed immobility group. It was first used to justify cyberbullying towards those who had to remain mobile within the community in the early phase of the pandemic and then absolve the self-motivated immobility group for their physical abuse that hindered the imposed immobility group from restoring mobility. Together, the self-motivated immobility group ignored the needs and attitudes of the imposed immobility people and deprived their rights of being in a state of security in the name of security.

Concluding Remarks

This chapter discusses two (im)mobility groups during the COVID-19 pandemic—the imposed immobility and the self-motivated immobility group. Results show that the imposed immobility group remained mobile within their communities while the self-motivated ones stayed at home in the dangerous days because the imposed mobility group did not have access to food and social activities they needed. Thereafter, the imposed immobility group did not restore their mobility until the lifting of the compulsory QR-code-for-buses policy in September while their self-motivated counterparts travelled as usual soon after the lifting of travel restrictions in late February.

The imposed immobility group had been in a state of insecurity throughout the pandemic. In the initial stage, they had to take the risk of infection to acquire daily necessities and fulfil their social needs outdoors. Furthermore, they had only insecure access to food, social interactions and social activities compared to the self-motivated ones even if they took the risk of infection. After the lifting of travel restrictions, they could not restore mobility due to their unfamiliarity with smartphones. They had been humiliated and abused by self-motivated people and therefore endured a state of insecurity caused by other people's claim for security.

Some results of this study, however, may not be transferrable to democratic contexts (see also Liu et al. 2020) since self-sacrifice for the country which has been widely propagated in authoritarian states (MacFarquhar 1974) is the philosophical underpinning of claiming staying at home as a patriotic behaviour. Nevertheless, this chapter is sufficiently clear that the human security approach can shed new insights into research on transport poverty and transport-related social exclusion.

References

Barter, P. A. (1999). Transport and urban poverty in Asia: A brief introduction to the key issues. *Regional Development Dialogue*, 20(1), 143–163.

Bureau of Statistics of Kunming. (2020). Statistical Communique of Kunming on the 2019 National Economic and Social Development. Retrieved from:

http://tjj.km.gov.cn/upload/resources/file/2020/05/09/3182042.pdf (in Chinese).

CHS (Commission on Human Security). 2003. *Human Security Now*. New York: Commission on Human Security.

Church, A., Frost, M., & Sullivan, K. (2000). Transport and social exclusion in London. *Transport Policy*, 7(3), 195–205.

Cicognani, E., Pirini, C., Keyes, C., Joshanloo, M., Rostami, R., & Nosratabadi, M. (2008). Social participation, sense of community and social well being: A study on American, Italian and Iranian university students. *Social Indicators Research*, 89(1), 97–112.

Domahidi, E., Breuer, J., Kowert, R., Festl, R., & Quandt, T. (2018). A longitudinal analysis of gaming-and non-gaming-related friendships and social support among social online game players. *Media Psychology*, 21(2), 288–307.

Farquhar, J., & Zhang, Q. (2012). *Ten thousand things: Nurturing life in contemporary Beijing*. Princeton: Princeton University Press.

Gatto, M., Bertuzzo, E., Mari, L., Miccoli, S., Carraro, L., Casagrandi, R., & Rinaldo, A. (2020). Spread and dynamics of the COVID-19 epidemic in Italy: Effects of emergency containment measures. *Proceedings of the National Academy of Sciences*, 117(19), 10484–10491.

Geurs, K. T., & van Wee, B. (2004). Accessibility evaluation of land-use and transport strategies: review and research directions. *Journal of Transport geography*, 12(2), 127–140.

Gilbert, M., Golding, N., Zhou, H., Wint, G. W., Robinson, T. P., Tatem, A. J., ... & Yu, H. (2014). Predicting the risk of avian influenza A H7N9 infection in live-poultry markets across Asia. *Nature communications*, 5(1), 1–7.

Handy, S. (2020). Is accessibility an idea whose time has finally come? *Transportation Research part D: Transport and Environment*, 83, 102319.

Huxhold, O., Miche, M., & Schüz, B. (2014). Benefits of having friends in older ages: Differential effects of informal social activities on well-being in middle-aged and older adults. *Journals of Gerontology Series B: Psychological Sciences and Social Sciences*, 69(3), 366–375.

Ishii-Kuntz, M. (1990). Social interaction and psychological well-being: Comparison across stages of adulthood. *The International Journal of Aging and Human Development*, 30(1), 15–36.

Kelly, M. E., Duff, H., Kelly, S., Power, J. E. M., Brennan, S., Lawlor, B. A., & Loughrey, D. G. (2017). The impact of social activities, social networks, social support and social relationships on the cognitive functioning of healthy older adults: a systematic review. *Systematic Reviews*, 6(1), 1–18.

King, G., & Murray, C. J. (2001). Rethinking human security. *Political Science Quarterly*, 585–610.

Krossbakken, E., Pallesen, S., Mentzoni, R. A., King, D. L., Molde, H., Finserås, T. R., & Torsheim, T. (2018). A cross-lagged study of developmental trajectories of video game engagement, addiction, and mental health. *Frontiers in Psychology*, 9, 2239.

Landstedt, E., & Persson, S. (2014). Bullying, cyberbullying, and mental health in young people. *Scandinavian Journal of Public Health*, 42(4), 393–399.

Lam, H. M., Remais, J., Fung, M. C., Xu, L., & Sun, S. S. M. (2013). Food supply and food safety issues in China. *The Lancet*, 381(9882), 2044–2053.

Litman, T. (2015). *Transportation affordability: Evaluation and improvements strategies*. Victoria, Canada: Victoria Transport Policy Institute.

Liu, Q., An, Z., Liu, Y., Ying, W., & Zhao, P. (2021a). Smartphone-based services, perceived accessibility, and transport inequity during the COVID-19 pandemic: A cross-lagged panel study. *Transportation Research Part D: Transport and Environment*, 97, 102941.

Liu, Q., Liu, Y., Zhang, C., An, Z., & Zhao, P. (2021b). Elderly mobility during the COVID-19 pandemic: A qualitative exploration in Kunming, China. *Journal of Transport Geography*, 96, 103176.

Liu, Q., Lucas, K., & Marsden, G. (2020). Public acceptability of congestion charging in Beijing, China: How transferrable are Western ideas of public acceptability? *International Journal of Sustainable Transportation*, 15(2), 97–110.

Liu, Q., Lucas, K., Marsden, G., & Liu, Y. (2019). Egalitarianism and public perception of social inequities: A case study of Beijing congestion charge. *Transport Policy*, 74, 47–62.

Lucas, K. (2006). Providing transport for social inclusion within a framework for environmental justice in the UK. *Transportation Research Part A: Policy and Practice*, 40(10), 801–809.

Lucas, K. (2012). Transport and social exclusion: Where are we now? *Transport Policy*, 20, 105–113.

Lucas, K. (2019). A new evolution for transport-related social exclusion research? *Journal of Transport Geography*, 81, 102529.

Lucas, K., Mattioli, G., Verlinghieri, E., & Guzman, A. (2016). Transport poverty and its adverse social consequences. *Proceedings of the Institution of Civil Engineers-Transport*, 169, 353–365.

MacFarquhar, R. (1974). *The origins of the Cultural Revolution: Volume II, the great leap forward 1958–1960*. New York: Columbia University Press.

Manion, M. (2014). *Retirement of revolutionaries in China: Public policies, social norms, private interests* (Vol. 258). Princeton: Princeton University Press.

Ministry of Health. (2003). Notification of SARS pandemic in China. Retrieved from: https://www.fmprc.gov.cn/web/ziliao_674904/zt_674979/ywzt_675099/zt2003_675963/2267_675979/t24141.shtml (in Chinese).

Mozur, P., Zhong, R., & Krolik, A. (2020). In Coronavirus fight, China gives citizens a color code, with red flags. *The New York Times*. Retrieved from: https://www.nytimes.com/2020/03/01/business/china-coronavirus-surveillance.html.

Nyqvist, F., Forsman, A. K., Giuntoli, G., & Cattan, M. (2013). Social capital as a resource for mental well-being in older people: A systematic review. *Aging & Mental Health*, 17(4), 394–410.

Riebel, J. R. S. J., Jäger, R. S., & Fischer, U. C. (2009). Cyberbullying in Germany—An exploration of prevalence, overlapping with real life bullying and coping strategies. *Psychology Science Quarterly*, 51(3), 298–314.

Rousseeuw, P. J. (1987). Silhouettes: A graphical aid to the interpretation and validation of cluster analysis. *Journal of Computational and Applied Mathematics*, 20, 53–65.

Salon, D., & Gulyani, S. (2010). Mobility, poverty, and gender: Travel 'choices' of slum residents in Nairobi, Kenya. *Transport Reviews*, 30(5), 641–657.

Sharifian, N., & Grühn, D. (2019). The differential impact of social participation and social support on psychological well-being: Evidence from the Wisconsin longitudinal study. *The International Journal of Aging and Human Development*, 88(2), 107–126.

Schwanen, T., Lucas, K., Akyelken, N., Solsona, D. C., Carrasco, J. A., & Neutens, T. (2015). Rethinking the links between social exclusion and transport disadvantage through the lens of social capital. *Transportation Research Part A: Policy and Practice*, 74, 123–135.

Thomas, D. R. (2006). A general inductive approach for analyzing qualitative evaluation data. *American Journal of Evaluation*, 27(2), 237–246.

Toker, S., & Baturay, M. H. (2016). Antecedents and consequences of game addiction. *Computers in Human Behavior*, 55, 668–679.

UNDP (United Nations Development Programme). 1994. *Human development report 1994: New dimensions of human security*. New York: Oxford University Press.

Velaga, N. R., Beecroft, M., Nelson, J. D., Corsar, D., & Edwards, P. (2012). Transport poverty meets the digital divide: Accessibility and connectivity in rural communities. *Journal of Transport Geography*, 21, 102–112.

Walker, G., & Day, R. (2012). Fuel poverty as injustice: Integrating distribution, recognition and procedure in the struggle for affordable warmth. *Energy Policy*, 49, 69–75.

Wei, W. (2014). With other people as mirror, you can see gain and lost clearly—Chinese elder people become bad or bad people grow old? *China-Today Forum*. (in Chinese).

Wu, F., Zhang, F., & Webster, C. (2013). Informality and the development and demolition of urban villages in the Chinese peri-urban area. *Urban Studies*, 50(10), 1919–1934.

Wu, H. L., Huang, J., Zhang, C. J., He, Z., & Ming, W. K. (2020). Facemask shortage and the novel coronavirus disease (COVID-19) outbreak: Reflections on public health measures. *EClinicalMedicine*, 21, 100329.

Xinhua News. (2020). Regional-, level-, category-based precision containment is implemented in Kunming. Retrieved from: http://www.yn.xinhuanet.com/newscenter/2020-02/21/c_138804374.htm (in Chinese).

Xue, J., & Zhang, W. (2013). Understanding China's food safety problem: An analysis of 2387 incidents of acute foodborne illness. *Food Control*, 30(1), 311–317.

Yang, H., Leung, C. B., Chen, H., & Liu, L. (2015). Privileged policies versus lack of care and engagement: The lives of retired veteran cadres in a residential community of Jinan Municipal Party Committee, China. *Asia Pacific Journal of Social Work and Development*, 25(4), 239–249.

Yang, Y. R., & Chang, C. H. (2007). An urban regeneration regime in China: A case study of urban redevelopment in Shanghai's Taipingqiao area. *Urban Studies*, 44(9), 1809–1826.

Zhong, X., & Chen, X. (2017). Demolition, rehabilitation, and conservation: Heritage in Shanghai's urban regeneration, 1990–2015. *Journal of Architecture and Urbanism*, 41(2), 82–91.

CHAPTER 7

Mental Health in the COVID-19 Pandemic and the Role of Social Media

Qian Zhang

When comparing the public's psychological responses to the COVID-19 epidemic with those in previous public health crises such as SARS and H1N1 breaks, one notable change is the increasingly essential role of digital technologies, particularly social media. Social media has been frequently used to obtain and share information during the COVID-19 epidemic, leading to the spread of both information and misinformation even faster than the virus itself. The social isolation in the physical world further increases the usage of social media as a main platform of social interactions, which may give a sense of connection or result in increased loneliness. The near-ubiquitous use of social media also provides valuable opportunities for researchers and professionals to understand and promote public mental health when conventional approaches are less feasible. Drawing from work on COVID-19 and previous public health

Q. Zhang (✉)
Independent Scholar, Beijing, China
e-mail: qzhangps@163.com

C. Zhang (ed.), *Human Security in China*,
https://doi.org/10.1007/978-981-16-4675-1_7

crises, this chapter gives an insight into the challenges and opportunities in public mental health during this unprecedented pandemic in the age of social media.

Psychological Responses and Mental Health During COVID-19 Pandemic in China

The COVID-19 pandemic is one of the most devasting catastrophes humans have experienced psychologically, of which the impact extends far beyond infected patients and healthcare workers. After the outbreak of the COVID-19 in late December 2019, Chinese researchers in mental health, psychology, psychiatry and public health made immediate efforts trying to gain a quick understanding of the Chinese public's psychological reactions and mental health status during the pandemic. According to a bibliometric analysis comparing mental health research in response to major global pandemics, China contributed to 12% of the total research output during COVID-19, ranking third of all states, despite the fact that 77% of the research output were from high-income countries (Maalouf et al. 2021). A reasonably large number of empirical studies have been conducted to investigate mental health aspects of the Chinese public during the COVID-19 pandemic, which is in sharp contrast to that of previous outbreaks such as SARS, H1N1 and Ebola. This can be primarily explained by the course and relative magnitude of the different outbreaks, considering COVID-19 was firstly reported in Wuhan and then rapidly transmitted across the country. The great research interest of Chinese academia also reflects the increasing attention of the governments and public institutions on public's mental health during public health crises. In addition, the advances in Internet technology and the popularity in social media have made such quick actions possible during the nationwide lockdown, as the majority of the empirical investigations have been conducted online, with many recruiting participants and collecting data through social media (Liu et al. 2020).

Public Psychological Responses to the COVID-19 Outbreak

Empirical research on the psychological impacts of COVID-19 has primarily documented the increasing symptoms of mental health distress, which might reflect a normative response to the extraordinary uncertainties and difficulties experienced by the public. Surveyed by psychiatrists at Shanghai Mental Health Centre, a nationwide large-scale survey conducted showed that by 10 February 2020, nearly 35% of the 52,730 respondents from 36 provinces, autonomous regions and municipalities in China experienced psychological distress (J. Qiu et al. 2020). Another study found that in a sample of 1210 Chinese citizens, 53.8% reported they experienced moderate-to-severe level of psychological effects during the first two weeks after the outbreak of the pandemic (Wang et al. 2020a).

Anxiety, depression and perceived stress were the most frequently observed immediate psychological reactions to the COVID-19 pandemic. Three online survey studies covering a total of 9610 citizens all over the country examined the prevalence of anxiety and depression symptoms among the general public in China during the initial stage (i.e. early January to mid-February 2020) of the pandemic (Ahmed et al. 2020; Huang and Zhao 2021; Wang et al. 2020a). Around one-third (29.0–36.4%) of the respondents reported experiencing anxiety, with around one in every five participants (18.9–28.8%) experiencing moderate-to-severe anxiety. Similarly, depression symptoms were experienced by 20.1–37.1% of the participants, and moderate-to-severe depression symptoms were found in 16.5–26.9% of the citizens. In addition, a survey study showed that in a sample of 1210 Chinese citizens, 32.1% experienced stress, of which 8.1% suffered from moderate-to-severe levels of perceived stress (Wang et al. 2020a). These findings are consistent with previous studies suggesting that anxiety, depression and stress were among the most profound psychological consequences of public health crises (Wong et al. 2007; Wu et al. 2005; Yu et al. 2005).

Usually, at early stages of a pandemic, the public lacks information about the nature, treatment, fatality rate, etc. of the newly emerging disease, resulting in a sense of uncertainty and fear. This is particularly the case for China. In the initial weeks after the outbreak, the governments and public health officials failed to release accurate and timely information about the epidemic. Meanwhile, both online and offline health information about COVID-19 was constantly censored by officials. These actions ignited negative emotional responses of the public. F. Hou and colleagues (2020) analysed social media data collected from three popular platforms in China from 1 December 2019 to 15 February 2020, revealing that anxiety, sadness and anger were the most frequently expressed public emotions related to COVID-19 on Sina Weibo (a microblogging platform). The expression of negative emotions peaked on 1 January, right after the Wuhan Municipal Health Commission announced a cluster of cases of viral pneumonia of unexplained aetiology; on 13 January, when the first confirmed cases abroad was reported; and on 6 February, when the whistle-blowing doctor Li Wenliang died from COVID-19. Notably, the expression of public anxiety declined steadily after the officials confirmed human-to-human coronavirus transmission on 20 January, while at the same time sadness and angry increased. These findings are consistent with another study applying the similar methodology and reporting a high volume of anxiety and confusion in Weibo posts by 20 January (Xu et al. 2020). However, according to Z. Hou et al. (2020), the public's negative emotions decreased gradually after containment measures were implemented by the government in late January.

The similar trend was also seen in survey studies. Several online survey studies were conducted between mid-February to March covering a total sample of 62,652 Chinese citizens showed lower prevalence rates of anxiety (13.3–31.6%) and depression (14.1–27.9%), especially moderate-to-severe anxiety (10.4–13.3%) and moderate-to-severe anxiety (10.8–18.8%), compared to that of the first several weeks (F. Hou et al. 2020; Ren et al. 2020; Shi et al. 2020; Wang et al. 2020b). In comparison, the prevalence rate of stress seemed to increase, with 67.9% (n = 809) reporting perceived stress (Ren et al. 2020) and 24.4% (n = 13,830) reporting an acute stress experience (Shi et al. 2020).

These changes in the public's emotional responses could partly be attributed to the government's actions. Despite the failure in providing sufficient and accurate information during the initial weeks, the Chinese government soon took actions to establish effective risk communication with the public. Overall, the Chinese government's outbreak communication has been more timely and transparent during COVID-19 compared to their response to the 2003 SARS outbreak (Liao et al. 2020). The public showed to be highly satisfied with the information they got during the pandemic (Tang and Zou 2021; Wang et al. 2020a), and showed a good level of the knowledge related to COVID-19 (Huang and Zhao 2021; Li et al. 2020; Lin et al. 2020a; Yue et al. 2021; Zhong et al. 2020). Such effective outbreak communication is suggested to relieve the public's fear and sense of uncertainty, and therefore reducing mental distress (Ren et al. 2020; Wang et al. 2020a, b; Q. Zhou et al. 2020). Meanwhile, the Chinese government imposed a series of prevention and control measures, including the nationwide lockdown, centred or home quarantine, limiting unnecessary public gathering and contact tracing. These measures proved to be effective in containing the spread of COVID-19 and exerted mixed impact on the public's mental health. The rapid and decisive containment measures provide the public a sense of security during the pandemic. Survey studies exploring the public's attitudes towards the pandemic showed that more than 90% of the respondents believed that the pandemic is controllable and China can win the battle with it (Yue et al. 2021; Zhong et al. 2020). The public showed a high compliance with containment measures and active engagement in preventive behaviours (Q. Chen et al. 2021; X. Wang et al. 2020). Complying with containment measures (e.g. home self-quarantine, social distancing) and preventive behaviours (e.g. wearing masks, frequently washing hands) were found to be associated with less mental health issues such as anxiety and depression (Lu et al. 2020; Ren et al. 2020; Wang et al. 2020b; Q. Zhou et al. 2020).

However, the lockdown and stay-at-home policies also caused substantial disturbance to people's daily lives, resulting in stress-induced changes to people's lifestyles and livelihood (Guo et al. 2020). S. X. Zhang et al. (2020) found that in a sample of 369 adults from 64 cities in China, 64.5% had to work from home or stop working during the early stage of the outbreak, and these participants reported higher levels of mental health problems compared to those who continued going to work at their office. Vulnerable groups including those with pre-existing mental disorders or chronic physical diseases, frontline workers, those in the most severely affected areas and those who are less financially well-off were more likely to be negatively affected by the quarantine (Wang et al. 2021). The increased sedentary time, decreased interpersonal communication and reduced income may also induce stress during the lockdown. The long-term impact of lockdown and quarantine on the public's mental health needs to be further investigated.

In addition to the major health mental problems summarised above, other common psychological reactions during the pandemic included posttraumatic disorder symptoms (PTSS) (7.0%; Ren et al. 2020), insomnia (18.2–29.2%; Huang and Zhao 2021; Shi et al. 2020) or clinical insomnia (5.7–7.2%; Ren et al. 2020; Shi et al. 2020), suicidal ideation (2.8%; Ren et al. 2020), and lower life satisfaction and subjective well-being (Ahmed et al. 2020; S. X. Zhang et al. 2020). Behavioural changes including increased smoking (30.1%) and alcohol consumption (11.3%) were also observed (Ren et al. 2020), which could be attributed to the elevated mental distress induced by the pandemic. Overall, the prevalence of the mental health symptoms during the pandemic was higher compared to that before the outbreak, during which the prevalence of depression, anxiety and insomnia was approximately 3.6%, 5.0% and 15.0%, respectively (Cao et al. 2017; Huang et al. 2019).

Despite the overall negative psychological consequences and mental health burden of the Chinese public, positive emotional and behavioural changes were also discovered in response to the COVID-19 outbreak. Two survey studies covering a total of 684 Chinese citizens found that more than half of the respondents (55.6–77.9%) reported they received increased support from their family and friends, were more likely to share feelings with others and showed increased caring for family members' feelings. They also showed higher levels of self-caring than before the pandemic, paying more attention to their mental health and spending more time in rest and relaxation (Cao et al. 2020; Zhang and Ma 2020). These positive responses may also contribute to the decreases in the public's negative sentiments over time.

Vulnerable Populations to the Pandemic's Psychological Impact

Some populations were found to be more psychologically vulnerable to the pandemic. Higher prevalence rates of psychological distress and mental health issues have been consistently observed in frontline healthcare workers (Huang and Zhao 2021; Liu et al. 2020; Shi et al. 2020), the elderly (J. Qiu et al. 2020; Q. Zhou et al. 2020), young people (Ahmed et al 2020; F. Hou et al. 2020; Huang and Zhao 2021; J. Qiu et al. 2020; Shi et al. 2020), and people with low levels of education (F. Hou et al. 2020; Wang et al. 2020a; Q. Zhou et al. 2020). Considering the highest mortality rate occurred among the elderly during the pandemic, it is not surprising that elderly people are more likely to be psychologically affected (J. Qiu et al. 2020). For young people, the high level of negative psychological outcomes has been attributed to social media exposure (J. Qiu et al. 2020; Shi et al. 2020). Although sufficient and timely information acquirement usually acts as a protective factor, excessive exposure to the pandemic-related information on social media, which is quite common among adolescents and young adults, can lead to elevated mental distress (Gao et al. 2020; Zhao and Zhou 2020; Zhang et al. 2021). People with lower levels of education are more likely to encounter difficulties in assessing credible sources and obtaining sufficient information, and therefore experiencing negative psychological consequences (Q. Zhou et al. 2020).

Notably, Zhou and colleagues (2020) found that farmers were the mostly affected group among all investigated occupations, indicating people of lower socioeconomic status could suffer more during the pandemic. Lacking access to public resources, their needs and well-being could be largely impacted and neglected (Horton 2020). In addition, as the majority of empirical investigations on public's mental health during COVID-19 have been conducted online via social media, those who have limited access to the Internet and social media are ruled out, leading to very little understanding of mental health status of this high-risk community and considerable bias in research outcomes.

The Role of Social Media

The COVID-19 pandemic occurred in an age of social media. For the Chinese general population under the strict "staying at home" policy, social media became a major way to communicate with the outside world. Evidence from empirical studies have shown a substantial increase in social media exposure and usage since the COVID-19 outbreak (Gao et al. 2020; Li et al. 2020). This section examined how the social media usage influenced the public's mental health during the COVID-19 in China, and particularly, investigated the public's psychological reactions to the government's actions as well as the pandemic through the lens of social media.

China's Social Media Environment and Ecosystem

The past decade has seen a tremendous rise of social media in China and its fundamental influence on daily life. Released by Tencent in 2011, WeChat (*Weixin*) has become China's dominant social media platform boasting more than 1.2 billion monthly users by the end of 2020 (Tencent 2020). It appears that WeChat has become ingrained into many Chinese people's daily life. People use it to send instant messages, make free phone calls, share pictures and videos and pay bills (Zhang et al. 2017). Sina Weibo is another major Chinese social media platform launched in 2009. Sina Weibo provides microblogging service, enabling users to send and receive short character-limited posts and retrieve textual content by searching for specific keywords. Sina Weibo represents the leading Chinese microblogging platform which attracts more than 5.1 million monthly users by September 2020 (Weibo 2021). Other popular social media platforms that have drawn researchers' attention to investigate the public's psychological responses during the COVID-19 in China include TikTok (*Douyin*), a video-sharing platform launched in 2016; and Baidu search engine, the largest search engine in China.

One unique feature of the social media ecosystem in China is the prevalent interventions by the government. Chinese Internet and its users are largely separated from the World Wide Web by the great firewall. Social media platforms are censored through blacklists keywords. Content containing blacklisted keywords cannot be posted on social media. The social media companies are also enforced to censor their content according to the government's guidelines. Content classified as sensitive are usually removed by social media platforms and the account posting such content could be suspended or closed. However, the official criteria for classifying sensitive content could be sometimes ambiguous to the public. The censorship system exerts significant influence on the public's social media engagement behaviour in China, which should be taken into consideration when drawing conclusions on social media data.

Social Media as a Crucial Source of Information and Misinformation

The outbreak of such unparalleled magnitude put the public in a highly uncertain situation that changed rapidly. To regain a sense of certainty and security, individuals usually create urgent and immense needs for reliable information and effective crisis communication (Liao et al. 2020). Studies conducted before the COVID-19 showed that social media including WeChat and Sina Weibo increasingly acted as important platforms for obtaining and sharing health information in China (Liu et al. 2017; Zhang et al. 2017). During the COVID-19, the role of social media in risk communication became even more significant.

An online survey study (Yue et al. 2021) investigating 517 Chinese urban and rural residents showed that 92.0% acquired information and knowledge related to COVID-19 primarily from social media, while TV is the only mentioned traditional media used by 66.2% of the respondents. Wang et al. (2020b) found that in a sample of 1304 Chinese citizens, 31.4% spent more than two hours per day viewing information about COVID-19 on social media at the early stage of the pandemic.

Chinese government across different levels also actively employ social media including Sina Weibo, WeChat and TikTok to disseminate information, facilitate the public's awareness and attitudes towards containment measures and prompt citizen engagement (Chen et al. 2020; Q. Chen et al. 2021). Chinese citizens usually accorded high credibility to such resources. For example, an interview study with a small group of residents in Hubei Province showed that the governments' verified social media accounts on Weibo and WeChat were the most often used and trusted information sources during the lockdown (Tan and Zou 2020). As discussed in the first section of this chapter, obtaining timely and accurate information from trusted sources effectively alleviate emotional distress during various stages of the pandemic (Lin et al. 2020b; Wang et al. 2020a, b).

However, excessive media exposure has been consistently associated with elevated mental distress during the pandemic (Gao et al. 2020; Zhao and Zhou 2020; Zhang et al. 2021). One possible explanation is that the frequent engagement in social media improves the risk for exposure to misinformation. Along with the rapid spread of the virus, a global epidemic of misinformation emerged. The COVID-19 epidemic is therefore labelled as an infodemic (Lancet Infectious Diseases 2020). Misinformation including rumors, fake news and conspiracy theories can be a natural by-product of any crisis. However, it poses new challenges during the COVID-19 pandemic, as misinformation spreads faster and further than ever in the age of social media (Zarorcostas 2020).

In China, the COVID-19 infodemic was even more serious. A study found that approximately 87% of social media users in China encountered COVID-19-related misinformation (Jiang 2020). Zhang and colleagues (2021) analysed a total of 19,188 original posts related to COVID-19 on major Chinese social media platforms from 20 January to 28 May, 2020, and identified 14.3% ($n = 2745$) of the posts as misinformation. Chat platforms (40.1%), video-sharing platforms (23.4%) and news-sharing platforms (22.1%) represented the major source of the misinformation. More misinformation was posted on the days when confirmed and suspected cases increased. The most frequently posted misinformation was about conspiracy theories (e.g. "Dr. Li Wenliang danced before his death"), followed by fake news and rumors related to government response (e.g. "Wuhan gas station would be closed"), prevention action (e.g. "Smoking vinegar can prevent the virus"), new cases, transmission route and origin and nomenclature (e.g. "COVID-19 is a biological weapon"), vaccines and medicines and symptoms and detection. The widespread misinformation can induce anxiety, panic and fear. By analysing data collected from Sina Weibo and Ali platform (a popular internet-based e-commerce marketplace in China), Z. Hou et al. (2020) found rumors and misinformation regarding prevention and treatment methods on social media, such as "Shuanghuanglian (a traditional Chinese herbal medicine for the treatment of cold and flu) and garlic can effectively prevent COVID-19", led to immediate panic buying. Individuals aged over 60 years, in lower socioeconomic groups, not working or not able to work and with more than two suspected symptoms were suggested to be more vulnerable to misinformation on social media (J. Zhou et al. 2020).

The Chinese government has taken a number of anti-online-rumor measures and collaborated with major social media companies in their efforts countering misinformation. Such efforts have been rightly more aggressive during the COVID-19 pandemic. Since late January, popular social media platforms, such as WeChat and Weibo, has initiated special rectification campaigns against the pandemic-related rumors. On 6 February, the Chinese government announced that spreading misinformation and rumors about COVID-19 can be punished as libel (China's Health Commission 2020). Misinformation and fake news have been removed swiftly, and the accounts posting such content shut down. An empirical study analysing COVID-19-related rumors on Sina Weibo showed that the official accounts of national authorities and local agencies responded to rumors very timely, usually debunking rumors within 1–2 days (B. Chen et al. 2021). Effective rumor control and clarification can alleviate the negative impacts of rumors and misinformation, improve the public's trust in government and enhance citizen's risk perception.

Meanwhile, under the strict censorship policy in China, rumors about public crisis can be highly politicised. For example, Li Wenliang, the whistle-blowing doctor who first warned the outbreak, was accused by police of spreading fake news before he was awarded with the May 4th Medal for his extraordinary contribution to the epidemic control. The censorship can significantly affect Chinese citizens' perception of misinformation and rumors. An interview study with 17 residents in Hubei Province revealed that when defining rumor, some of the participants primarily considered if the information was approved by the government or could lead to public panic (Zou and Tang 2021). Participants also showed mixed and slightly contradictory attitudes towards the information/misinformation on social media (Tang and Zou 2021). On one hand, almost all participants expressed high levels of trust in and satisfaction with the COVID-19-related information authorised by the government. Some participants believed the government would effectively debunk misinformation and rumors they encountered on social media. Such perceptions and attitudes could produce a sense of security and certainty in an infodemic. On the other hand, they were aware of the censorship and actively engaged in self-censorship, knowing some information could be removed for political reasons, and being more cautious when sharing such information, which seemed to reveal a sense of insecurity using social media.

Social Media for Emotional Expression and Social Support

The protective effect of emotional expression and social support in mental health has been well documented (Kane et al. 2019; Morelli et al. 2015). COVID-19 has been such a stressful period during which individuals may sometimes or consistently feel helpless and overwhelmed. To maintain good levels of psychological functioning and well-being, it is essential to appropriately express their feelings and get emotional support from others. However, the nationwide lockdown along with quarantine and stay-at-home policies have largely reduced in-person interactions. Therefore, social media has been acting as the main platform for such psychological needs.

Several studies analysing Weibo and WeChat content found that during the early stage of the pandemic, the public made very quick responses to the spread of the disease and government actions on social media, and expressed a wide range of emotions accordingly (Z. Hou et al. 2020; Li et al. 2020; Liao et al. 2020; J. Wang et al. 2020; Xu et al. 2020). The most frequently expressed emotion was anxiety (Z. Hou et al. 2020; Li et al. 2020; Xu et al. 2020), which is inconsistent with evidence from survey studies cited in the first section of this chapter. Other emotions widely expressed included sad, fear, worry, concern, anger, indignation and blame. For example, Li et al. (2020) found the public expressed increased concern about health, death and family after the confirmation of human-to-human transmission. Liao et al. (2020) discovered a frequent expression of blame towards individuals who put others at greater risk as well as government, particularly local government agencies for their perceived failures in risk communication and control measures. Z. Hou et al. (2020) revealed that the death of Dr. Li Wenliang renewed the public's expression of anger. Positive emotional expressions were also observed, such as empathy, hope, optimism, faith, blessing, contentment and praise (Li et al. 2020; Liao et al. 2020; J. Wang et al. 2020). The public on social media showed empathy towards those in the most affected areas and lacked access to medical resources, and praised front-line healthcare workers for their contribution and sacrifice. Engaging in discussions about the pandemic and related public events on social media can not only act as an emotional outlet, but also provide individuals a sense of unity and connection.

Moreover, social media also become an important channel for social support. Luo et al. (2020) found many individuals turned to Sina Weibo for both instrumental and emotional support during the pandemic, and identified a total of 9826 posts on Weibo between January and May 2020 as seeking support. Interestingly, they found that those support-seeking posts expressing anger rather than fear or sadness received the most reposts. These posts usually showed angry about hospitals' unfair treatment or official institutions' delayed responses. Those who reposted these posts echoed these feelings, showed empathy towards the help seekers and urged relevant departments to take effective measures. A survey study involving 320 Wuhan residents showed that Wuhan residents gained a significant amount of emotional and peer support from WeChat during the lockdown, which had beneficial effects on stress management and behavioural change (Zhong etal. 2021). Guo et al. (2021) found that the public were more likely to interact with the posts on official government social media accounts showing emotional rather than instrumental support. These findings highlight the importance of social support, especially emotional support, from social media during the COVID-19 pandemic.

Social Media for Mental Health Services

As reviewed above, the COVID-19 pandemic induced wide-ranging impacts on the public's mental health, which could be more profound than previous public health crises such as SARS and H1N1, considering its unprecedented magnitude. However, one significant difference from previous public health crises happened in China is that timely mental health services were initiated and implemented shortly after the outbreak of COVID-19 (N. Zhang et al. 2020). As early as 24 January, 2020, just one day after the lockdown implementation of Wuhan, the Wuhan Mental Health Centre launched the first free crisis intervention hotline of mental health to the public. Later, the National Health Commission of China (NHC) released several guideline documents, addressing the importance of psychological crisis intervention as an integral part of the public health response to the COVID-19, and urging immediate actions of and effective collaboration between mental health associations, academic societies and multidisciplinary mental health teams. Theory- and evidence-based psychological crisis interventions and psychoeducation were soon developed, mainly targeting vulnerable populations including frontline healthcare workers, infected and suspected patients on quarantine sites, those living in high-prevalence areas and those with serious mental health (Peng et al. 2020).

Meanwhile, social media becomes the major platform for mental health services targeting the general public. National and provincial psychology organisations rapidly launched psychoeducation programmes and self-help materials. More than 40 books, hundreds of popular science articles and numerous audio/video tutorials have been published targeting various population groups with different levels of mental health needs, freely available on WeChat, Weibo and TikTok (Ju et al. 2020). Online psychological counselling services have also been widely established by mental health professionals and academic societies throughout the country, providing free 24-h services on WeChat. In addition, psychological self-help intervention systems and artificial intelligence programmes were also used via social media to tackle public mental health issues (Liu et al. 2020).

Overall, the COVID-19 has seen a great progress of China's emergency interventions in the aspects of mental health, which is enabled by the near-ubiquitous use of social media. Governmental agencies, academic societies and mental health professionals have been working together proactively to enhance the general public mental health during the unprecedented pandemic. Various forms of individual-centred and evidence-based psychological interventions were established, aiming at improving psychological resilience and well-being of the general public. Nevertheless, there remains limitations and challenges for China's mental health support during COVID-19. Despite the wide-ranging interventions and programmes launched, to date there is a lack of solid empirical evidence specifying the acceptability, feasibility and effectiveness of the interventions for their targeting populations, which is though understandable due to the rapid evolution of the epidemic. Some scholars have raised concern about the potential low awareness and utilisation of mental health services (Ju et al. 2020; D. Qiu 2020; Yao et al. 2020). In addition, online services via social media may exacerbate health disparities, in that a significant digital divide still exists in China (Yao et al. 2020). Further steps are needed to increase the public's awareness and usage, establish evidence base and improve socioeconomic equity in mental health services.

Conclusions

This chapter gives a summary of Chinese public's psychological responses and mental health during the COVID-19 pandemic based on existing empirical evidence, and highlights the role of social media. Firstly, social media was used as an important tool for researchers and professionals to investigate the public's psychological responses immediately after the outbreak of COVID-19. High prevalence rates of mental health symptoms including anxiety, depression and perceived stress were observed among the general public. The containment measures implemented by the government exerted mixed impacts on the public's mental health, which decreased anxiety and depression by effectively controlling the pandemic, but could cause substantial disturbance to people's daily lives and induce long-term stress. Secondly, social media served as a platform of effective risk communication during the pandemic. Chinese citizens obtained pandemic-related information primarily from social media, and showed a high level of trust and satisfaction of the information released by government officials. Obtaining sufficient information from credible resources helped the citizens maintain a sense of control and alleviate mental distress. Meanwhile, COVID-19-related misinformation and rumors spread across social media, inducing anxiety, fear and panic buying among the public. The government's censorship on social media information may cause contradictory sentiments in such an infodemic. Moreover, social media has been used as a channel for emotional expression and social support. The social media users gained a sense of connection during the lockdown by expressing opinions and emotions towards the pandemic, the government's actions and others. Finally, social media provided opportunities for mental health services, enabling a great progress of China's emergency interventions in the aspects of mental health. A wide range of psychological interventions and mental health support have been launched on social media, of which the feasibility and effectiveness remain to be examined.

References

Ahmed, M. Z., Ahmed, O., Aibao, Z., Hanbin, S., Siyu, L., & Ahmad, A. (2020). Epidemic of COVID-19 in China and associated psychological problems. *Asian Journal of Psychiatry, 51*, 102092. https://doi.org/10.1016/j.ajp.2020.102092.

Cao, Y., Ma, Z. F., Zhang, Y., & Zhang, Y. (2020). Evaluation of lifestyle, attitude and stressful impact amid COVID-19 among adults in Shanghai, China. *International Journal of Environmental Health Research*. https://doi.org/10.1080/09603123.2020.1841887.

Cao, X-L., Wang, S-B., Zhong, B-L., Zhang, L., Ungvari, G. S., Ng., C. H., Li, L., Chiu, H. F. K., Lok, G. K. I., Lu, J-P., Jia, F-J., & Xiang, Y-T. (2017). The prevalence of insomnia in the general population in China: A meta-analysis. *PloS ONE, 12*(2), e0170772. https://doi.org/10.1371/journal.pone.0170772.

Chen, B., Chen, X., Pan, J., Liu, K., Xie, B., Wang, W., Peng, Y., Wang, F., Li, N., & Jiang, J. (2021). Dissemination and refutation of rumors during the COVID-19 outbreak in China: Infodemiology study. *Journal of Medical Internet Research, 23*(2), e22427. http://www.jmir.org/2021/2/e22427/.

Chen, Q., Min, C., Zhang, W., Ma, X., & Evans, R. (2021). Factors driving citizens engagement with government TikTok accounts during the COVID-19 pandemic: Model development and analysis. *Journal of Medical Internet Research, 23*(2), e21463. https://doi.org/10.2196/21463.

Chen, Q., Min, C., Zhang, W., Wang, G., Ma, X., & Evans, R. (2020). Unpacking the black box: How to promote citizen engagement through government social media during the COVID-19 crisis. *Computers in Human Behavior, 110*, 106380. https://doi.org/10.1016/j.chb.2020.106380.

Chen, D., Song, F., Tang, L., Zhang, H., Shao, J., Qiu, R., Wang, X., & Ye, Z. (2021). Quarantine experience of close contacts of COVID-19 patients in China: A qualitative descriptive study. *General Hospital Psychiatry, 66*, 81–88. https://doi.org/10.1016/j.genhosppsych.2020.07.006.

China's Health Commission. (2020). *The opinions on punishing criminal and illegal activities that hinder the prevention and control of novel coronavirus pneumonia*. Available at http://www.nhc.gov.cn/xcs/pfzs/202002/6090ed34d8e64d038fbed94b9f957059.shtml.

Gao, J., Zheng, P., Jia, Y., Chen, H., Mao, Y., Chen, S., & Dai, J. (2020). Mental health problems and social media exposure during COVID-19 outbreak. *Plos One, 15*(4), e0231924. https://doi.org/10.1371/journal.pone.0231924.

Guo, J., Feng, X. L., Wang, X. H., & van IJzendoorn, M. H. (2020). Coping with COVID-19: Exposure to COVID-19 and negative impact on livelihood predict elevated mental health problems in Chinese adults. *International Journal of Environmental Research and Public Health, 17*, 3857. https://doi.org/10.3390/ijerph17113857.

Guo, J., Liu, N., Wu, Y., & Zhang, C. (2021). Why do citizens participate on government social media accounts during crises? A civic voluntarism perspective. *Information & Management, 58*, 103286. https://doi.org/10.1016/j.im.2020.103286.

Horton, R. (2020). Offline: 2019-nCoV—"A desperate plea." *Lancet, 395*, 400. https://doi.org/10.1016/S0140-6736(20)30299-3.

Hou, F., Bi, F., Jiao, R., Luo, D., & Song, K. (2020). Gender differences of depression and anxiety among social media users during the COVID-19 outbreak in China: A cross-sectional study. *BMC Public Health, 20*, 1648. https://doi.org/10.1186/s12889-020-09738-7.

Hou, Z., Du, F., Jiang, H., Zhou, X., & Lin, L. (2020). Assessment of public attention, risk perception, emotional and behavioural responses to the COVID-19 outbreak: Social media surveillance in China. *Preprints with The Lancet*. https://doi.org/10.2139/ssrn.3551338.

Huang, Y., Wang, Y., Wang H., et al. (2019). Prevalence of mental disorders in China: A cross-sectional epidemiological study. *The Lancet Psychiatry, 6*(3), 211-224. https://doi.org/10.1016/S2215-0366(18)30511-X.

Huang, Y., & Zhao, N. (2021). Mental health burden for the public affected by the COVID-19 outbreak in China: who will be the high-risk group? *Psychology, Health & Medicine, 26*(1), 23–24. https://doi.org/10.1080/13548506.2020.1754438.

Jiang, S. Infodemic: Study on the spread of and response to rumors about COVID-19 [in Chinese]. (2020). *Studies on Science Popularization, 15*(1), 70–78. https://doi.org/10.19293/j.cnki.1673-8357.2020.01.011.

Ju, Y., Zhang, Y., Wang, X., Li, W., Ng, R. M. K., & Li, L. (2020). China's mental health support in response to COVID-19: Progression, challenges and reflection. *Globalization and Health, 16*, 102. https://doi.org/10.1186/s12992-020-00634-8.

Kane, H. S., Wiley, J. F., Schetter, C. D., & Robles, T. F. (2019). The effects of interpersonal emotional expression, partner responsiveness, and emotional approach coping on stress responses. *Emotion, 19*(8), 1315–1328. https://doi.org/10.1037/emo0000487.

Li, S., Wang, Y., Xue, J., Zhao, N., & Zhu, T. (2020). The impact of COVID-19 epidemic declaration on psychological consequences: A study on active weibo users. *International Journal of Environmental Research and Public Health, 17*(6), 2032. https://doi.org/10.3390/ijerph17062032.

Liao, Q., Yuan, J., Dong, M., Yang, L., Fielding, R., & Lam, W. W. T. (2020). Public engagement and government responsiveness in the communications about COVID-19 during the early epidemic stage in China: Infodemiology study on social media data. *Journal of Medical Internet Search, 22*(5), e18769. https://doi.org/10.2196/18796.

Lin, Y., Hu, Z., Alias, H., & Wong, L. P. (2020a). Knowledge, attitudes, impact, and anxiety regarding COVID-19 infection among the public in China. *Frontiers in Public Health, 8*, 236. https://doi.org/10.3389/fpubh.2020.00236.

Lin, Y., Hu, Z., Ailas, H., & Wong, L. P. (2020b). Influence of mass and social media on psychobehavioral responses among medical students during the downward trend on COVID-19 in Fujian, China: A cross-sectional study. *Journal of Medical Internet Research, 22*(7), e19982. https://doi.org/10.2196/19982.

Liu, X., Lu, J., & Wang, H. (2017). When health information meets social media: Exploring virality on Sina Weibo. *Health Communication, 32*(10), 1252–1260. https://doi.org/10.1080/10410236.2016.1217454.

Liu, S., Yang, L., Zhang, C., Xiang, Y-T., Liu, Z., Hu, S., & Zhang, B. (2020). Online mental health services in China during the COVID-19 outbreak. *The Lancet Psychiatry, 7*(4), E17–E18. https://doi.org/10.1016/S2215-0366(20)30077-8.

Luo, C., Li, Y., Chen, A., & Tang, Y. (2020). What triggers online help-seeking retransmission during the COVID-19 period? Empirical evidence from Chinese social media. *PLoS ONE, 15*(11), e0241465. https://doi.org/10.1371/journal.pone.0241465.

Maalouf, F. T., Mdawar, B., Meho, L. I., & Akl, E. A. (2021). Mental health research in response to the COVID-19, Ebola, and H1N1 outbreaks: A comparative bibliometric analysis. *Journal of Psychiatric Research, 132*, 198–206.

Morelli, S. A., Lee, I. A., Arnn, M. E., & Zaki, J. (2015). Emotional and instrumental support provision interact to predict well-being. *Emotion, 15*(4), 484–493. https://doi.org/10.1037/emo0000084.

Peng, D., Wang, Z., & Xu, Y. (2020). Challenges and opportunities in mental health services during the COVID-19 pandemic. *General Psychiatry, 33*. E100275. https://doi.org/10.1136/gpsych-2020-100275.

Qiu, D., Li, Y., Li, L., He, J., Ouyang, F., & Xiao, S. (2020). Policies to improve the mental health of people influenced by COVID-19 in China: A scoping review. *Frontiers in Psychiatry, 11*, 588137. https://doi.org/10.3389/fpsyt.2020.588137.

Qiu, J., Shen, B., Zhao, M., Wang, Z., Xie, B., & Xu, Y. (2020). A nationwide survey of psychological distress among Chinese people in the COVID-19 epidemic: Implications and policy recommendations. *General Psychiatry, 33*, e100213. https://doi.org/10.1136/gpsych-2020-100213.

Ren, Y., Qian, W., Li, Z., Liu, Z., Zhou, Y., Wang, R., Qi, L., Yang, J., Song, X., Zeng, L., & Zhang, X. (2020). Public mental health under the long-term influence of COVID-19 in China: Geographical and temporal distribution. *Journal of Affective Disorders, 277*, 893-900. https://doi.org/10.1016/j.jad.2020.08.045.

Shi, L., Lu, Z-A., Que, J-Y., Huang, X-L., Liu, L., Ran, M-S., Gong, M., Yuan, K., Yan, W., Sun, Y-K., Shi, J., Bao, Y-P., & Lu, L. (2020). Prevalence of and risk factors associated with mental health symptoms among the general population in China during the Coronavirus Disease 2019 pandemic. *JAMA Network Open, 3*(7), e2014053. https://doi.org/10.1001/jamanetworkopen.2020.14053.

Tang, L., & Zou, W. (2021). Health information consumption under COVID-19 lockdown: An interview study of residents of Hubei province, China. *Health Communication, 36*, 1. https://doi.org/https://doi.org/10.1080/10410236.2020.1847447.

Tencent. (2020). *Tencent announces 2020 fourth quarter and annual results.* Available at https://static.www.tencent.com/uploads/2021/03/24/b83f5784d0579b51cf8515cf560b4256.pdf.

The Lancet Infectious Diseases, Editorial. (2020). The COVID-19 infodemic. *The Lancet Infectious Diseases, 20*(8), 875. https://doi.org/10.1016/S1473-3099(20)30565-X.

Wang, C., Pan, R., Wan, X., Tan, Y., Xu, L., Ho, C. S., & Ho., R. C. (2020a). Immediate psychological responses and associated factors during the initial stage of the 2019 Coronavirus Disease (COVID-19) epidemic among the general population in China. International *Journal of Environmental Research and Public Health, 17*, 1729. https://doi.org/10.3390/ijerph17051729.

Wang, C., Pan, R., Wan, X., Tan, Y., Xu, L., McIntyre, R. S., Choo, F. N., Tran, B., Ho., R., Sharma, V. K., & Ho., C. (2020b). A longitudinal study on the mental health of general population during the COVID-19 epidemic in China. *Brain, Behavior, and Immunity, 87*, 40-48. https://doi.org/10.1016/j.bbi.2020.04.028.

Wang, X., Lin, L., Xuan, Z., Xu, J., Wan, Y., & Zhou, X. (2020). Risk communication on behavioral responses during COVID-19 among general population in China: A rapid national study. *Journal of Infection, 81*, 911-922. https://doi.org/10.1016/j.jinf.2020.10.031.

Wang, Y., Shi, L., Que, J., Lu, Q., Liu, L., Lu, Z., Xu, Y., Liu, J., Sun, Y., Meng, S., Yun, K., Ran, M., Lu, L., Bao, Y., Shi, J. (2021). The impact of quarantine on mental health status among general population in China during the COVID-19 pandemic. *Molecular Psychiatry*. https://doi.org/10.1038/s41380-021-01019-y.

Wang, J., Zhou, Y., Zhang, W., Evans, R., & Zhu, C. (2020). Concerns expressed by Chinese social media users during the COVID-19 pandemic: Content analysis of Sina Weibo microblogging data. *Journal of Medical Internet Research, 22*(11), e22152. http://www.jmir.org/2020/11/e22152/.

Weibo. (2021). *The 2020 Weibo user development report*. Available at https://data.weibo.com/report/reportDetail?id=456.

Wong, T. W., Gao, Y., & Tam, W. W. S. (2007). Anxiety among university students during the SARS epidemic in Hong Kong. *Stress and Health, 23*, 31-35. https://doi.org/10.1002/smi.1116.

Wu, K. K., Chan, S. K., & Ma, T. M. (2005). Posttraumatic stress after SARS. *Emerging Infectious Diseases, 11*(8), 1297–1300. https://doi.org/10.3201/eid1108.041083.

Yao, H., Chen, J-H., & Xu, Y-F. (2020). Rethinking online mental health services in China during the COVID-19 epidemic. *Asian Journal of Psychiatry, 50*, 102015. https://doi.org/10.1016/j.ajp.2020.102015.

Yu, H. Y. R., Ho, S. C., So., K. F. E., & Lo, Y. L. (2005). The psychological burden experienced by Hong Kong midlife women during the SARS epidemic. *Stress and Health, 21*(3), 177–184. https://doi.org/10.1002/smi.1051.

Yue, S., Zhang, J., Cao, M., & Chen, B. (2021). Knowledge, attitudes and practices of COVID-19 among urban and rural residents in China: A cross-sectional study. *Journal of Community Health, 46*, 286–291. https://doi.org/10.1007/s10900-020-00877-x.

Xu, Q., Shen, Z., Shah, N., Cuomo, R., Cai, M., Brown, M., Li, J., & Mackey, T. (2020). Characterizing Weibo social media posts from Wuhan, China during the early stages of the COVID-19 pandemic: Qualitative content analysis. *JMIR Public Health and Surveillance, 6*(4), e24125. http://publichealth.jmir.org/2020/4/e24125/.

Zarorcostas, J. (2020). How to fight an infodemic. *The Lancet, 395*, 676. https://doi.org/10.1016/S0140-6736(20)30461-X.

Zhang, Y., Li, R., Sun, X., Peng, M., & Li, X. (2021). Social media exposure, psychological distress, emotion regulation, and depression during the COVID-19 outbreak in community samples in China. *Frontiers in Psychiatry, 12*, 644899. https://doi.org/10.3389/fpsyt.2021.644899.

Zhang, Y., & Ma, Z. F. (2020). Impact of the COVID-19 pandemic on mental health and quality of life among local residents in Liaoning Province, China: A cross-sectional study. *International Journal of Environmental Research and Public Health, 17*, 2381. https://doi.org/10.3390/ijerph17072381.

Zhang, S. X., Wang, Y., Rauch, A., & Wei, F. (2020). Unprecedented disruption of lives and work: Health, distress and life satisfaction of working adults in

China one month into the COVID-19 outbreak. *Psychiatry Research, 288*, 112958. https://doi.org/10.1016/j.psychres.2020.112958.

Zhang, X., Wen, D., Liang, J., & Lei, J. (2017). How the public uses social media WeChat to obtain health information in China: A survey study. *BMC Medical Informatics and Decision Making, 17*(66), 71–79. https://doi.org/10.1186/s12911-017-0470-0.

Zhang, N., Wu, K., & Wang, W. (2020). Timely mental health services contribute to the containment of COVID-19 pandemic in China. *Global Health Research and Policy, 5*, 40. https://doi.org/10.1186/s41256-020-00168-x.

Zhao, N., & Zhou, G. (2020). Social media use and mental health during the COVID-19 pandemic: moderator role of disaster stressor and mediator role of negative affect. *Applied Psychology: Health and Well-Being, 12*(4), 1019–1038. https://doi.org/10.1111/aphw.12226.

Zhong, B., Huang, Y., & Liu, Q. (2021). Mental health toll from the coronavirus: Social media usage reveals Wuhan residents' depression and secondary trauma in the COVID-19 outbreak. *Computers in Human Behavior, 114*, 106524. https://doi.org/10.1016/j.chb.2020.106524.

Zhong, B-L., Luo, W., Li, H-M., Zhang, Q-Q., Liu, X-G., Li, W-T, & Li, Y. (2020). Knowledge, attitudes, and practices towards COVID-19 among Chinese residents during the rapid rise period of the COVID-19 outbreak: A quick online cross-sectional survey. *International Journal of Biological Science, 16*(10), 1745–1752. https://doi.org/10.7150/ijbs.45221.

Zhou, J., Ghose, B., Wang, R., Wu, R., Li, Z., Huang, R., Feng, D., Feng, Z., & Tang, S. (2020). Health perception and misconception regarding COVID-19 in China: Online survey study. *Journal of Medical Internet Research, 22*(11), e21099. https://doi.org/10.2196/21099.

Zhou, Q., Hu, Z., Bian, G., Yu, H., Li, X., Lu, Y., Yu, C., Li, X., Yao, Q., Zhou, W., Yuan, T-F., & Zhou, D. (2020). Mental health and psychological function of general population during the COVID-19 epidemic in China. *Clinical and Translation Medicine, 10*(2), e103. https://doi.org/10.1002/ctm2.103.

Zou, W., & Tang, L. (2021). What do we believe? Rumors and processing strategies during the COVID-19 outbreak in China. *Public Understanding Science, 30*(2), 153-168. https://doi.org/10.1177/0963662520979459.

CHAPTER 8

Health Security and Public Health Emergency Management in China

Jia Liu

This article discusses public health emergency management in China from the perspective of health security. Drawing on the ideas of securitization theories, China's responses to Covid-19 were characterized as processing from "a-securitization" to "hyper-securitization". This article explains the legal and institutional structure operating behind the a-securitization and hyper-securitization processes. The a-securitization occurred against China's legal inconsistencies and fragmented "*tiao-kuai*" institutions; however, when strong leadership was provided by the top leaders of the Communist Party, the Covid-19 combat demonstrated features of hyper-securitization, which were made possible by the flexibility and responsiveness of China's legal system and the patterns of governance to overcome bureaucratic and hierarchical fragmentation. It suggests that

J. Liu (✉)
Institute of Public Policy (IPP), South China University of Technology, Guangzhou, China
e-mail: liujia@scut.edu.cn

C. Zhang (ed.), *Human Security in China*,
https://doi.org/10.1007/978-981-16-4675-1_8

while the hyper-securitization measures may have effectively curbed the state-level outbreaks, they have also disproportionately increased the panic of citizens.

Health-Security Linkage: Securitization and Public Health Emergency Management

Few emerging infectious diseases have posed such vital challenges to the world so quickly and dramatically as Covid-19. As of this writing, the worldwide transmission of Covid-19 is widespread, calling for immediate and decisive public health emergency management. Given that a large number of people are under a serious threat across the world, many countries have declared an entrance of a constitutional state of emergency or a state of public health emergency. Public health emergency management addresses hazards and vulnerabilities whose timing, unpredictability or scale threatens to overwhelm routine capabilities (Nelson et al. 2008). To provide immediate and decisive responses to the Covid-19 outbreak, governments need to exercise emergency powers and actions that may not wait for deliberation under ordinary constitutional rule. During the Covid-19 outbreak, some governments around the world, including the Chinese government, have been perceived as "moved along the a-securitization to hyper-securitization gamut" (Stivas and Sliwinsk 2020). How did China respond to Covid-19 along with the processes from "a-securitization" to "hyper-securitization"? How did such a public health emergency issue become securitized in China? What were the legal and institutional mechanisms operating behind the processing from the process of a-securitization to the process of hyper-securitization?

In the post-Cold War era, to highlight that many non-traditional security issues were developed into security threats, securitization theories proposed alternatives to the framework of considering a security issue through realist lenses as a self-evident one. To explain the processes of how non-traditional security issues were securitized, grounded in constructive perspectives, the Copenhagen School of securities theories led by Barry Buzan, Ole Wœver, Jaap de Wilde, and others outlined the process of framing an issue as a security threat and providing a policy reaction to the perceived threat (see Buzan et al. 1998). When public health issues were increasingly seen as security issues, political scientists further explored the linkages between health and security. In the 1980s, when the spread of HIV/AIDS was perceived as a threat to security, the linkage between health and security was established by revealing the devastating impacts of HIV on armed forces and the stability of fragile states (Elbe 2011, 850–851). During the SARS outbreak, however, the linkage between health and security issues was established due to "the mortality it caused and because of its potentially very serious economic repercussions" (ibid., 851). In the age of globalization, SARS was perceived as a threat that "could spread rapidly around the planet and wreak havoc on the world economy" (ibid.). Thus, unlike the HIV/AIDS construed as a threat to the state, the SARS was rather perceived as a threat to the world population and the resulting severe world economic disruptions. Moreover, when the emergence of the H5N1 influenza pandemic was perceived as a security concern, it was not due to its high morbidity and mortality but because of the economic effects. This was because H5N1 could not sustain rates of human-to-human transmissions as high as SARS, but "the lingering spectre of an imminent H5N1 pandemic [] compelled them to remain vigilant about the prospect of a new pandemic erupting unexpectedly at any moment, and to engage in a plethora of pandemic preparedness activities". Thus, the emergence of H5N1 further broadened the scope of health insecurity to encompass the threats posed by the infectious diseases that may have the potential of a future outbreak (ibid.).

The securitization theories thus have provided a useful tool to outline the stages of the responses to the outbreak of a public health emergency. In Western contexts, how is a threat framed as a security issue? According to securitization theories, a security issue was declared by political actors as an existential threat. Threats are framed as security issues by identifying and declaring particular referent objects as existential threats to security. The process of threat identification is followed by acceptance of the securitization of the issue by a specific target audience. The declaratory speech act of identifying the issue as a threat is a securitizing move, which does not create securitization, while the securitization of the issue is created when the target audience accepts as such (Lo 2015, 5). The audience's acceptance further leads to a shift from normal measures to emergency ones (Buzan et al. 1998, 26). The securitization theories thereby identify three core elements of securitization—i.e., "speech acts", "emergency measures" and "audience acceptance". From their standpoint, the securitization is "self-referential" in nature, because it "mean[s] the issue is presented as an existential threat, requiring emergency measures and justifying actions outside the normal bounds of political procedure" (ibid., 23–24). The securitization theories emphasize the power of language in shifting an issue into a security threat rather than identifying a real threat issue. Given the self-referential nature of the security issue, its scope can be extended beyond traditional military problems to encompass transnational crimes, migration, infectious diseases, such as HIV/AIDS, SARS, H5N1 and Covid-19.

In non-Western contexts, given that processes and measures of securitization may demonstrate different features, the preceding analytical framework needs to be revised. Writing of the AIDS pandemic as a threat to national security in China and India, Catherine Yuk-Ping Lo proposes a revised framework of securitization in non-Western, non-democratic contexts. She cautiously reminds us of holding the view of seeing security as a binary division. As echoed by Vuori as well as McInnes and Rushton, securitization possesses "a continuum of success and failure" (Lo 2015, 24). Through incorporating ideas from public policy research, she suggests that "a securitizing move (speech acts plus emergency measures) resembles the policy formulation and policy decision-making stage" and "[t]he process of acceptance is similar to the stage of policy evaluation" (ibid., 26). She thus categorizes the three core elements of securitization theories—i.e., speech acts, emergency mode/measures and audience acceptance—further into positive and negative speech acts, subcategories of emergency measures and different types of audience (ibid., 27–36).

In light of the preceding ideas and inspirations, it is crucial to locate health security in the context of China. As David Fidler once commented, "China still looms large in any future confrontation with SARS, raising concerns about China's attitude should the virus and disease return. As a group of public health experts observed, '[m]any of the solutions to solve the multifaceted puzzle of SARS and to prevent future epidemics must come from China'" (Fidler 2004, 190). China's suppressing the debate on political reform after the SARS outbreak creates worries and fears about whether China will provide transparent and timely responses to the outbreak of novel diseases. In this sense, China's engagement with Covid-19—a prominent challenge—provides us with a crucial touchstone to examine China's legal and institutional structure of securitizing the epidemics.

Moreover, given that the term of "security" is not a concept without contestation, the concept of health security is similarly contested. While the terms of national security and human security may not be mutually distinguishable and transferable, they have different implications for understanding regarding "whose security is under at risk". National security is often conceptualized in this manner—that is, "the referent object of security is the state; that the main concerns are direct threats, usually military in nature" (McInnes 2015, 8). National security's linkage with health is established due to the former's concern with the physical condition of the military troops. When the traditional focus of national security on military troops is gradually expanded to encompass a larger range of risks, such as the risks caused by an increased global movement of goods, services and people, the linkage between health and national security is further expanded to include the risks of infectious diseases to economic growth and international stability (ibid.).

By contrast, the concept of human security focuses on individuals. The ascendance of human security is captured in a series of UN documents, in particular the UN Development Program's 1994 Human Development Report on "New Dimensions of Human Security" and the 2003 Commission on Human Security Report, "Human Security Now: Protecting and Empowering People". The 1994 Human Development Report outlines the key areas of human security, i.e., economic security, health security, food security, personal security, environmental security, community security and political security. Apart from recognizing the key areas, it also highlights four characteristics essential to human security, i.e., (1) it is a universal concern, (2) its components are interdependent, (3) it is better ensured through earlier prevention than later intervention, and (4) it is people-centered (UNDP 1994, 23–24). At the core of human security lies the shift of security's focus from the state to the people. As stated by the 1994 UNDP Report, security.

> has for too long been interpreted narrowly: as security of territory from external aggression, or as protection of national interests in foreign policy. . . . Forgotten were the legitimate concerns of ordinary people who sought security in their daily lives. . . . For many of them, security symbolized from the threat of disease, hunger, unemployment, crime, social conflict, political repression and environmental hazards. . . . For most people, a feeling of insecurity arises more from worries about daily life than from the dread of a cataclysmic world event. (ibid., 22)

From this standpoint, what the concept of human security aims to achieve is emancipator and normative in nature, depicting "the world can and should be run in a different, better way by putting people first" (McInnes 2015, 12). The world that highlights human security focuses on two key aspects: freedom from fear and freedom from want. Starting with each individual's health condition, the concept of human security further suggests that "improved health may lead to economic growth as people become better able to work and less dependent upon health services" (ibid.). Economic growth and social stability in turn benefit health security through reducing fears from want.

Thus, this chapter examines the legal and institutional structure of public health management to respond to the Covid-19 outbreak from the perspective of the securitization theories. In light of the analytical distinctions between national security and human security, this chapter also analyzes whether the a-securitization and hyper-securitization responses to the Covid-19 outbreak were constructed in terms of more traditional national stability, social stability, and economic development, or in terms of human security, freedom from want and freedom from fear. Following this section, the second section briefly describes the initial responses of the local governments of Wuhan and Hubei towards the Covid-19 outbreak and explains how institutional and legal structure was operated behind the responses. The third section aims to outline the measures employed in order to combat the Covid-19 after the central government securitized the issue and discuss the legal and institutional structure operating behind the measures. The chapter concludes with that while the hyper-securitization measures may have effectively curbed the community-level outbreak, they have also disproportionately increased the panic of citizens, exacerbating the human security of Chinese citizens.

A-Securitization: Legal and Institutional Structure

In December 2019, a mysterious disease was reported to be found at a hospital in the city of Wuhan, the capital city of Hubei Province. The cause of the pneumonia was later found to be a new coronavirus, known as SARS-CoV-2. While as of the writing, China has effectively controlled the spread of the disease, at the initial stage of the Covid-19 outbreak the local governments of Hubei and Wuhan were criticized for their late responses to prevent and control the spread of the disease. The initial stage of the local governments' response was described as a-securitizing the COVID-19 outbreak—which denotes "a condition where important social phenomena are declared security irrelevant" (Sliwinski 2016, 25)—for the purpose of soothing the panic of Chinese citizens and keeping the economy running (Stivas and Sliwinsk 2020). This section identifies the local Wuhan and Hubei governments' initial responses to the Covid-19 outbreak and explains the legal and institutional structure operating behind their responses.

The first case of the unknown pneumonia was reported to be detected in Wuhan Jinyintan Hospital on December 1, 2020. By December 8, more cases with unknown causes were found in the South China Seafood Market. The local medical workers reported the emergence of the unknown disease to the Wuhan Center for Disease Control and Prevention. Huang Chaolin, the vice president of Jinyintan Hospital also published a paper in the Lancet, suggesting that "there may be human-to-human transmissions, but it is hard to conclude due to the small number of cases" (Liu et al. 2020, 204). By the end of December, however, due to the limited knowledge of the Covid-19, the Health Commission of Wuhan reported that there was "no evidence of significant human-to-human transmission" (ibid., 203). Since the beginning of January 2020, when the first group of experts arrived at Wuhan for an investigation, they isolated the virus, obtained the entire genetic sequence and submitted it to the World Health Organization; however, they still considered the disease as "preventable and controllable" (ibid., 204). On January 15, the Wuhan Municipal Health Commission announced that "there is no clear evidence of human-to-human transmission"; however, it did not deny "the possibility of limited human-to-human transmission" and claimed that "the risk of continuous human-to-human transmission is low" (ibid., 205). Despite this, the Wuhan local government did not cancel the "Ten-Thousand Family Reunion Banquet" held on January 18 (ibid.). Moreover, despite the increasingly huge number of suspicious cases, the early warning of whistleblowers (including the late Dr. Li Wenliang) failed to motivate the local governments to issue a warning for the public or to take systematic precautionary actions until the evidence of human-to-human transmission was confirmed on January 20, after Zhong Nanshan, a well-known expert in respiratory diseases was sent to Wuhan for an investigation on January 19. The Chinese local governments' initial responses to Covid-19 were thus widely criticized as ineffective and untimely (see *South China Morning Post* 2020; *The Guardian* 2020).

Why did the local governments of Wuhan and Hubei fail to take active and decisive actions, for instance, to issue an early warning for the general public at the initial stage of the Covid-19 outbreak?

The legal and institutional structure of the Chinese government contributed to the belated responses from the local governments. The legal framework of public health emergency management was constituted by numerous laws and regulations. The core legal documents were the Law on the Prevention and Treatment of Infectious Diseases (hereinafter "PCID") which was adopted in 1989 and revised respectively in 2004 and 2013, the Law on Emergency Response adopted in 2007 and the Regulation on Handling Public Health Emergencies issued by the State Council immediately after the SARS outbreak in May 2003.

While the three legal documents set out the legal framework of China's public health emergency management, there were inconsistencies between them, which were an important factor contributing to the delayed early warning made by the local governments. The Law on Emergency Response establishes a bottom-up emergency reporting system. With respect to who is legally mandated to inform the outbreak of an unknown disease to the public, according to the Law on Emergency Response, the local governments at or above the county levels are responsible for reporting to the governments at the higher levels; they also ought to timely and regularly release the information related to the emergencies to the public.[1] Thus, the Wuhan Municipal Government is responsible for reporting information regarding the epidemic to its superiors and releasing the related information to the public according to the Law on Emergency Response.

In contrast, however, the 2013 PCID adopts a top-down management system. According to the 2013 PCID, the MOH (the current "National Health Commission", hereinafter "NHC") is mandated to regularly and timely release information regarding the nation-scope epidemic situations of infectious diseases to the public, and it is also allowed to authorize the health departments at the provincial level to publish information on the epidemic situations of infectious diseases within their administrative regions.[2] Thus, while the Hubei Provincial Government was authorized to publish information regarding the epidemic to the public, the

[1] See Article 44 of the Law on Emergency Response.

[2] See Article 38 of the PCID.

Wuhan Municipal Government could only do this after it obtained authorization from the Provincial Government. The inconsistencies between the two statutes caused problems in implementation. From the legal perspective, it was unclear who was legally authorized to release the information regarding the emergency outbreak, which gave rise to the problem that the governments of Wuhan and Hubei did not release information regarding the outbreak of the unknown disease to the public.

Moreover, the institutional structure behind the legal inconsistencies, which was called by scholars as *tiao-tiao/kuai-kuai* and the resulting pattern of a dual rule, also perplexed the situation. In a recently published article, Jacques DeLisle and Kui Shen gave an explanation for China's initial delayed responses to the Covid-19. As explained by them, officials at departments of sub-national levels in China have to be responsible for two masters—"'vertically' to superiors in a functionally defined, hierarchical bureaucratic structure that reaches up to a ministry (or similar central entity) in Beijing (for which the metaphor is *tiao*—a long, narrow piece); and 'horizontally' to the general-purpose government at the official's own level—provincial, municipal, or still-lower (for which the analogy is *kuai*—a 'lump' or block)" (DeLisle and Shen 2021, 25).

The *tiao* and *kuai* approaches to addressing public health emergency management, however, are supported by different rationales. The *tiao* approach emphasizes opinions and judgements of expertise in the field of public health, which adopts the measure, among others, of providing experts early access to information and the authority to make informed judgements when the outbreak of a serious infectious disease threatens (ibid.). Some elements of the PCID focus on *tiao*. The PCID gives the NHC and its local health commissions the powers and obligations to manage the work of prevention, treatment and control of infectious diseases. The Law on Emergency Response and the related regulations also adopt elements emphasizing *tiao*. For instance, the Law on Emergency Response assigns tasks to the NHC of developing emergency response plans and establishing criteria for each of the four-level public health emergencies. Pursuant to the regulations related to public health emergencies, the NHS and local health commissions also have functions and obligations to dispatch experts to access public health emergencies, determine the categories of emergencies and notice lower-level public health authorities of the existence of such an emergency (ibid., 27).

The *kuai* approach, however, emphasizes the functions and obligations of local officials to monitor, guide and coordinate the work of local-level branches of public health and medical agencies. Responsibility for negative outcomes of the public health and medical work is also undertaken by local officials (ibid., 25–26). The key elements of the Law on Emergency Response focus on *kuai*. The obligations and functions of preparing, detecting, declaring, informing and responding to public health emergencies are allocated to local-level governments (starting from the county level) within the jurisdiction covering an affected area. The emergency response system is tiered with each level of government responsible to report to the higher-level government during the outbreak of an emergency (ibid., 26). The PCID also has provisions emphasizing *kuai*. Each level of government is assigned with the responsibility of guiding the prevention and control work of public health emergencies and receiving reports from the Health Commission and the CCDC of the same level (ibid.).

In an ideal situation, *kuai* approach allows a clear allocation of responsibility to each particular level of government, avoiding the problem of "passing the buck upward". The *tiao* approach enables a rapid reporting system to the central political leaders, helping to bypass the delays of information reporting and emergency approvals. In the public health system, however, the *tiao* was dominated by *kuai* in the sense that the behaviors of officials of the vertical functional lines were given priority to the officials of the territorial units (Yang 2020). CDC was more close to a department responsible for technical supervision (Yang 2020; Li et al. 2020). Moreover, the officials of local territorial units may report to superiors as required by the PCID, but the reporting may not yield positive effects for them. This is because for local officials it is unclear whether the uncertain disease is serious or not. If it is simply a fleeting problem, the avoidance of which may not be seen as a significant effort and the reporting of which to higher authorities may be regarded as shirking responsibility. The officials' disclosure to the public may even cause panic in society and resulting harm to local economic and socially important activities (DeLisle and Shen 2021, 29). Yet on the other hand, if local officials keep silent information about the emerging yet not serious problem, they may resolve it by themselves without letting higher-level authorities and the public know about it. However, if the unreported issue proves unmanageable, the failure of local governments to promptly report may cause severe sanctions (ibid.).

In China's initial response to the Covid-19 outbreak, the local governments of Wuhan and Hubei tended to cover up the unknown disease.

When a novel coronavirus was reported to be found, the Wuhan Health Commission issued two notices to local medical institutions regarding the discovery of a new disease, but it did not disclose the information to the public (Wei et al. 2020). When the experts of the NHC arrived at Wuhan, Wuhan local officials and administrators of medical institutions withheld information suggesting human-to-human transmissions. As complained by a member of the second expert team, "we didn't see a formal report, including how the disease came about, how it was discovered, what investigations were done, what the investigation results were, which cases were first discovered... We didn't have any knowledge of these. Later we did not have any other ways, so basically we were only in charge of clinical treatments" (Yu and Li 2020). Moreover, according to this member, local Wuhan officials and administrators of medical institutions directed the public health and medical work under the "principle of local management" [shudi guanli] (DeLisle and Shen 2021, 26). However, when the local Wuhan officials played the dominant role of managing the unknown disease, it seems that they gave priority to the local conditions of social stability and economic development when it was scientifically uncertain whether the disease was severe or not (Liu et al. 2020, 204).

It is a given that Covid-19 poses a significant challenge to the health security and human security of individuals. Not only must an individual ensure the physical burden of such a disease, but one has to also endure its potential side effects and associated socioeconomic burdens. Unlike ordinary infectious diseases, such as seasonal influenza, HIV/AIDS, malaria, etc., however, dealing with the emergence of a novel disease is involved with uncertainty, in the sense that "[w]e respond to the likelihood of death in the event the disease is contracted, rather than the compound probability of contracting the disease and succumbing to its effects" (Stern 2002, 105). The uncertainty involved with responding to the disease often generates panic disproportionate to the disease-caused mortality. Moreover, an unknown disease is often associated with isolation, social distancing, wide fear and restrictions on commerce and international trade (Huang 2013, 83). In this sense, there are additional unknown socioeconomic consequences of the novel disease beyond the level of the health security of individual sufferers. Such aggregated effects may further challenge state capacity and regime security, including the state's ability to deliver public healthcare services and effectively make the economy running. The indirect costs of an emerging novel disease—such as the loss of productivity and work and the loss of public trust towards the regime—were well recognized by the Chinese central and local governments after the SARS outbreak. As one official was reported to have commented, SARS was a "huge shock for the entire party, you can sense this at internal meetings, where the atmosphere has changed and people are expressing criticisms more freely. The SARS epidemic is forcing us to rethink the whole theoretical framework for government that was developed under Jiang Zemin" (Saich 2006, 103). Thus, considering that restrictions imposed by a government may be counterproductive, the government may face a dilemma between whether to publish information regarding the epidemic and to take decisive and immediate actions at the initial stage of the outbreak. This might be the consideration of the Chinese local governments of Wuhan and Hubei which tended not to disclose the epidemic information to the general public. Moreover, the initial belated responses of the local governments of Wuhan and Hubei were largely a-securitized, which was operated in a legal and institutional environment of the inconsistency of the core public health laws and regulations as well as ambiguity born of the *tiao-kuai* bureaucratic fragmentation.

Hyper-Securitization: Legal and Institutional Structure

After recognizing that Covid-19 was the "most challenging public health emergency" the state has encountered after its founding in 1949, Xi highlighted that "[l]ife is of paramount importance" on January 20 (Xinhua News 2020). On the same day, Premier Li Keqiang in an executive meeting of the State Council decided to take steps for the prevention and control of the epidemic (State Council Information Office). A central leading group on the epidemic response was established on January 25, which was decided at the meeting of the Standing Committee of the Central Political Bureau of the Communist Party. As said by Xi, "[w]hatever situations it encounters or whatever needs it has, the group can directly phone me" (Xinhua News 2020). After the securitizing move was made, swift and decisive extraordinary measures were taken, which involved travel restrictions, tracing, testing, isolation and treatment of infected people, and mass deployment of personal protective equipment under the state of a public health emergency. The responses at this stage were characterized as "hyper-securitization" (Stivas and Sliwinsk 2020). This section explains how the securitizing move was made, what kind of extraordinary measures was taken and how the mechanisms were operated allowing the hyper-securitization measures to be taken in response to the Covid-19 outbreak in China.

The Copenhagen School believes that securitizing actors—who perform the speech act of security—are collectivities or designated authoritative representatives, such as states, parties or pressure groups, etc. In China, however, it was the top leaders of China who recognized the urgency of the Covid-19 outbreak and made the securitizing move. On January 20, Present Xi Jinping gave important instructions on the prevention and control of the epidemic, highlighting the priority of the life and health of citizens (Xinhua News 2020). Xi urges that a "people's war" should be launched to fight against this "invisible enemy" (ibid.). Moreover, in the Chinese context, "security" is translated as *anquan*, but *anquan* in Chinese denotes "safety" rather than "security". Equivalent and related terms may be used to express security acts, such as "great problem", "tremendous problem" and "serious problem" (Lo 2015, 29). Thus, as an authoritarian state, China's securitization of threats is used as an effective means of elevating the particular issue on the national agenda.

After the top leader recognized the significance of this issue, a series of extraordinary measures were taken. For instance, on January 23, a critical decision of the lockdown of Wuhan was made. After the disease spread to Hong Kong and other provinces across China, all 31 provinces of mainland China launched the highest-level responses to public health emergencies by January 29 (Caixin 2020). The elements of the response playbook, such as travel restrictions, tracing, testing, isolation and treatment of infected people, and mass deployment of personal protective equipment, were also incorporated into prevention and control measures in China. What was the legal and institutional structure operating behind effectively taking this set of extraordinary measures?

First, integrative mechanisms were used to bind the fragmented hierarchical governments and ministries. Meetings were convened to bring together officials from hierarchical systems and diverse localities (Lieberthal and Oksenberg 1988, 151–160). During different stages of the Covid-19 combat, Xi made response demands at a great number of high-level meetings, such as 17 meetings of the Standing Committee of the Political Bureau of the CPC Central Committee and four meetings of the Political Bureau of the CPC Central Committee (Xinhua News 2020). Moreover, the Central Leading Group for Prevention and Control of Covid-19 (hereinafter "CLG") was established to coordinate the activities of different commissions and ministries and to provide personnel, material, and financial resources. The CLG was headed by the Premier, which was composed of senior political members of the Communist Party of China Politburo and the State Council. It issued "directives [that] were considered as uncompromisable political tasks to be fulfilled by participants" (He et al. 2020, 246). The Central Steering Group for Prevention and Control of Covid-19 (hereinafter "CSG") was also established as the CLG's representative to supervise the combat Covid-19 on the front line in Hubei Province. To facilitate interdepartmental coordination, the CSG was composed of 11 ministerial-level cadres (Sohu News 2020). Parallel epidemic prevention and control headquarters were also established in different regions across China to coordinate the activities of lower-level commissions and ministries.

Under the guidance of the CLG, functional boundaries between commissions and ministries as well as the geographical boundaries between provinces could be overcome. For instance, NHC, the Ministry of Transportation, the Ministry of Industry and Information Technology, the Ministry of Education, the military, the Supreme Court, and other related organs, as well as their local departments were all mobilized to prevent the further spread of the disease (DeLisle and Shen 2021, 44). Enormous administrative regulations were enacted by the central-level commissions and ministries since the lockdown of Wuhan on January 23. 536 documents were issued as Covid-19 countermeasure-related documents released by the related departments (see chart 1).[3] On the interpretative level, the Supreme People's Court issued notices and announcements. They included, in the area of civil, commercial and economic law, intellectual property tribunal on the arrangements for legal proceedings and litigation services,[4] intellectual property tribunal on the arrangement for online case filing and mailing of case-filing materials,[5]

[3] 536 documents on infectious disease prevention and control were issued by the central government departments between January 24, 2020 and January 1, 2021. Source: Compiled by the author from the feature column in PKULaw (access January 4, 2021).

[4] Announcement of the Intellectual Property Tribunal of the Supreme People's Court on the Arrangements for Legal Proceedings and Litigation Services during the Prevention and Control of the Covid-19 Outbreak, "最高人民法院知识产权法庭关于疫情防控期间诉讼活动、诉讼服务工作安排的公告," January 29, 2020.

[5] Announcement of the Intellectual Property Tribunal of the Supreme People's Court on Matters concerning Online Case Filing and Mailing of Case-filing Materials during the

the enforcement work,[6] online litigation,[7] judicial departments legally ensuring the resumption of work and production,[8] three notices on hearing civil cases[9] and travel contract disputes resolution (Table 8.1).[10]

Second, from formal laws and regulations to ad hoc measures, the Chinese central and local governments' innovation and use of the dynamic aspects of the Chinese legal system were pervasive. In response to the epidemic most countries passed new laws and issued new policies to meet the urgent needs of the changing situations of the public health emergency. The declaration of entering into a constitutional state of emergency allowed many governments to make exceptions to the existing legal rules and patterns of governance (Coglianese and Mahboubi 2021). In China,

Prevention and Control of the Covid-19 Outbreak, "最高人民法院知识产权法庭关于新型冠状病毒感染的肺炎疫情防控期间网上立案、邮寄立案事宜的公告," January 29, 2020.

[6] Notice by the Enforcement Bureau of the Supreme People's Court of Matters concerning Effectively Conducting the Enforcement Work during the Period of Prevention and Control of the Outbreak of Novel Coronavirus Pneumonia, "最高人民法院执行局关于做好防控新型冠状病毒肺炎疫情期间执行工作相关事项的通知," January 30, 2020.

[7] Notice by the Supreme People's Court of Strengthening and Regulating the Online Litigation Work during the Period of Prevention and Control of the Covid-19 Outbreak, "最高人民法院关于新冠肺炎疫情防控期间加强和规范在线诉讼工作的通知," February 14, 2020.

[8] Notice by the CPC Political and Legislative Affairs Committee, the Supreme People's Court, and the Supreme People's Procuratorate of Issuing the Opinions on Procuratorial, Judicial and Public Security Departments Legally Ensuring the Resumption of Work and Production during the Epidemic Prevention and Control, "中共中央政法委员会、最高人民法院、最高人民检察院等关于印发《关于政法机关依法保障疫情防控期间复工复产的意见》的通知", February 25, 2020.

[9] Notice by the Supreme People's Court of Issuing the Guiding Opinions (Part I) on Several Issues of Properly Hearing Civil Cases concerning the COVID-19 Pandemic, "最高人民法院印发《关于依法妥善审理涉新冠肺炎疫情民事案件若干问题的指导意见（一）》"; Notice by the Supreme People's Court of Issuing the Guiding Opinions (Part II) on Several Issues of Properly Hearing Civil Cases concerning the COVID-19 Pandemic, "最高人民法院印发《关于依法妥善审理涉新冠肺炎疫情民事案件若干问题的指导意见（二）》"; Notice by the Supreme People's Court of Issuing the Guiding Opinions (Part III) on Several Issues of Properly Hearing Civil Cases concerning the COVID-19 Pandemic, "最高人民法院印发《关于依法妥善审理涉新冠肺炎疫情民事案件若干问题的指导意见（三）》".

[10] Notice by the Supreme People's Court, the Ministry of Justice and the Ministry of Culture and Tourism of Legally and Properly Resolving Travel Contract Disputes involving the COVID-19 Pandemic, "最高人民法院、司法部、文化和旅游部关于依法妥善处理涉疫情旅游合同纠纷有关问题的通知".

Table 8.1 Chart 1 (Data collected from PKULaw)

Commissions and Ministries	*Total*
National Health Commission (卫生健康委员会)	64
Ministry of Transport (交通运输部)	53
Ministry of Finance (财政部)	48
Ministry of Civil Affairs (民政部)	34
Ministry of Commerce (商务部)	33
Ministry of Human Resource and Social Security (人力资源和社会保障2021 部)	30
Ministry of Education (教育部)	23
State Administration for Market Regulation (国家市场监督管理总局)	21
State Taxation Administration (国家税务总局)	18
National Development and Reform Commission (国家发展和改革委员会)	17
Ministry of Agriculture and Rural Affairs (农业农村部)	16
Ministry of Housing and Urban and Rural Development (住房和城乡建设部)	14
Others	204

however, while the Covid-19 was perceived as a security issue, a constitutional state of emergency was not invoked.[11] The whole-of-government and whole-of-society measures were effectively taken under the state of a public health emergency—that is, the highest level of emergency was invoked in accordance with the Law on Emergency Response below the constitutional state of emergency and the most severe level of infectious diseases (Type A restrictions) according to the PCID was invoked.

Under the state of a public health emergency, local governments were innovative in using the flexibility in the form of laws and regulations. For instance, the lockdown measures were taken by local governments of Wuhan and other municipalities through issuing notices. The notice issued by Zhangwan District, Shiyan City provided that wartime control measures would be implemented from February 12, 2020 (Sina Net 2020). It specified that "from 24:00 on February 12, Zhangwan District will implement wartime control" (ibid.). The alleged "wartime control

[11] According to Article 67(20) of the P. R. China Constitution, the Standing Committee of the National People's Congress exercises the function and power of deciding that the whole country or individual provinces, autonomous regions and municipalities enter into a state of emergency. Article 89 (16) stipulates that the State Council has the power to decide some areas within provinces, autonomous regions and municipalities to enter into a state of emergency.

measures" were not legally authorized. The power to legally declare an entrance into the constitutional state of emergency is empowered to the Standing Committee of the National People's Congress and the State Council in China. The local governments of Wuhan and other municipalities were not legally empowered by the Constitution to make such a declaration. Moreover, sometimes it was an over-reaction to the local epidemic situations. Some of the wartime measures were not de facto necessary. Wuhan was the place where the epidemic was most severely hit by the Covid-19 outbreak. In Hubei, the epidemic in Shiyan was not as urgent as in Wuhan and Xiaogan. As of 12:00 on February 14, the number of confirmed cases in Hubei Province was 51,986. Among the 17 cities, Shiyan had a total of 586 confirmed cases, ranking 12th in the province. The wartime control notice was promulgated after full deliberation and discussion with local residents in Zhangwan District, but this notice was not reported to the Epidemic Prevention and Control Headquarters in Shiyan City before its promulgation (ibid.). To the extent that the local government's notice was made after the deliberation, it was not only a rhetoric acknowledgment of the seriousness of the epidemic, but also a performative action of its firm determination to take decisive actions to combat the epidemic.

The discretion of the local administrative agencies was made possible by the vagueness of China's laws and regulations. For instance, Article 42 of the PCID endows the discretionary power on taking prevention and control measures to local governments at county or above levels; the measures include restricting gathering activities, suspension of work, enclosing water and food sources, closure of the places that may cause the spread of the infectious diseases, etc. However, the PCID does not specify the circumstances under which it is necessary to take the aforementioned measures. Article 42 of the PCID specifies that "[i]n the event of an outbreak or epidemic of an infectious disease, the local people's governments at or above the county level shall immediately organize forces to carry out prevention and control in accordance with the prevention and control plan, cut off the transmission of the infectious disease, report to the higher-level people's government for decision, and may take emergency measures when necessary". In this situation, local administrative agencies are forced to interpret the legislation and issue rules regarding the necessary conditions that allow the preceding extraordinary measures to be taken. To combat the Covid-19 outbreak, Wuhan's lockdown was decided by the Wuhan Prevention and Control Headquarter. The Wuhan

Prevention and Control Headquarter successively issued two executive notices, No. 1 and No. 2 Notices for the Prevention and Control of the Covid-19 outbreak. The notices demanded that the city's buses, subways, ferries, and long-distance transportations should be suspended; citizens should not be allowed to leave Wuhan and Wuhan railway stations and airports should be temporarily closed. In this sense, during the outbreak of an uncertain novel virus, "[n]ations require nimble legal dynamism not merely because of the novelty of this particular virus itself, but also because the behaviors, attitudes, and interests of individuals within society are themselves so varied and changing" (Coglianese and Mahboubi 2021, 10). In China, while the state did not enter into the constitutional state of emergency, the local governments were still empowered to take advantage of the flexibility in the legal system to issue executive notices. The source of the flexibility was from the vagueness of the specification of the Chinese laws and regulations.

Third, during the Covid-19 outbreak, some weaknesses of the Chinese legal system which were constraints in other countries were conducive to China's combat against the Covid-19 outbreak. In China, while privacy and privacy rights were valued by some Chinese people, especially the urban younger generation, when the centrally demanded measures were taken, the discontents felt by ordinary people were not transformed into lawsuits to challenge the surveillance tracking notices (DeLisle and Shen 2021, 49). During the Covid-19 outbreak, mass surveillance, intelligence tracking, data collection, internet censorship and social credit systems were all used to monitor and detect breaches of public health and safety directives (Houston 2020). Some cyber surveillance and data collection measures were conducted even before the risks to public health and safety had been proved. Chinese citizens were encouraged to install the QR code system which allowed governmental authorities to know whether they had been exposed to the virus of the Covid-19. This system was enabled by a nationwide telecom data analysis platform under the Ministry of Information Industry Technology after the Covid-19 outbreak. This platform allowed three major telecom carriers of China (China Mobile, China Telecom and China Unicom) to provide a tracking record of citizens' locations in the past 15 or 30 days (Norton Rose Fulbright 2020). According to the notice issued by the Cyber-Security Administration of China, entities authorized by the NHC were permitted to collect data without seeking consent from citizens (ibid.). While both the government and private sectors authorized by the government might have access to personal data, the legal regulation for the possession, use, and storage of the data lacked transparency.

While discontents might have been felt by ordinary citizens towards some extremely rigorous quarantine mandates and isolation orders, their discontents could not be developed into lawsuits to challenge the legality of those rigorous measures and to prevent their effective implementation. In the Chinese context, the laws and regulations require that local governments exercise discretionary power in an appropriate manner. For instance, Article 11 of the Law on Emergency Response stipulates that "The emergency response measures taken by a relevant people's government and its departments shall be appropriate for the nature, degree, and extent of the social damage caused by an emergency incident; and where multiple measures are available for selection, those conducive to the maximum protection of the rights and interests of citizens, legal persons, and other organizations shall be selected". This Article requires a proportionality test of the benefits and harms of the measures taken to each individual's rights and interests, including the condition of human security. As noted earlier, during the period of Wuhan's lockdown, Zhangwan District government also issued a notice to implement the lockdown measures. These measures were taken by the local governments which were endowed with the discretionary power by the laws and regulations; however, in circumstances where confirmed cases, suspected cases, and close-contact cases had been identified and isolated, if the local governments still implemented the lockdown notices, these measures would be inappropriate in the sense that they might have disproportionately increased the panic of individual citizens. In this sense, the Chinese legislation indeed requires a consideration of the human security of each individual citizen, in particular the health security in the sense of protecting the people's freedom from fear.

Although the Chinese legislation has recognized this, the judicial review of administrative rules and actions has not been actively and prevalently taken in China. For instance, there was a recent case in which Madeng sued the Huidong County Forest Public Security Bureau.[12] It was reported that during the fire prohibition period in Huidong County, the plaintiff used her portable lighter to burn mulberries at the edge of the forest area without getting authorization or approval. The

[12] Sichuan Case No. 3426 in 2019,[(2019) 川3426行初11号].

defendant, Huidong County Forest Public Security Bureau, decided to impose an administrative penalty of 10 days of administrative detention on the plaintiff in accordance with Article 50(1)(1) of the Public Security Administration Punishment Law, which specifies that those who refuse to implement the decisions and orders issued by the people's governments in a state of emergency will be imposed a warning or a fine of not more than 200 *yuan*, and under serious circumstances detention may be imposed for not less than 5 days but not more than 10 days as well as a fine of not more than 500 *yuan*. The plaintiff believed that the defendant simply identified the forest fire prohibition period in Huidong County as a state of emergency. She also mentioned that the Standing Committee of the National People's Congress and the State Council had not declared an entrance into a constitutional state of emergency, and the Constitution did not authorize county-level governments to make decisions and to declare an entrance of an emergency. The plaintiff thus filed an administrative lawsuit in front of the Court of Huidong County. After hearing the arguments of both sides, the Court held that the state of emergency includes a constitutional state of emergency and public health emergencies, ecological disasters, accidents, economic crisis and public safety incidents within the jurisdictions at local levels. As the Court also put it, the constitutional state of emergency at the national level was stipulated in the Constitution, while the state of emergency at the local levels not only referred to an "emergency" that had occurred, but included the risks that had to be regulated and avoided. The Court further clarified the distinction between a constitutional state of an emergency and a de facto state of an emergency—that is, in this case the understanding of an emergency suggested by the plaintiff was a constitutional state of an emergency, while the state of emergency applied by the local county government was a de facto one. Thus, the Court decided that the notice issued by the local public security bureau was not illegal because the sanctions created by the notice were within the scope of the discretionary power and the authority endowed by the Public Security Administration Punishment Law. In this sense, to the extent that administrative litigation has only very limited effectiveness, citizens may not effectively challenge the legality of the administrative actions and rules in China. Although the limited effectiveness of judicial review has been seen as a weakness of the Chinese legal system for a long time, during the Covid-19 outbreak the weakness in turn guaranteed the operation of the executive orders issued by multiple levels of governments.

By taking advantage of the dynamics and flexibility of the legal system, the Chinese governments effectively countered the spread of the disease. On March 31 it was announced by the Chinese government that large-scale domestic transmission of the disease was stopped. On April 8 the 76-day outbound traffic restrictions of Wuhan were eased, and local daily life and work started to return to normal. During the hyper-securitization process, however, while the local governments effectively curbed the community-level spread of Covid-19 through taking some rigorous measures, some of the measures might have brought about disproportionate harms to individual citizens. To the extent that the judicial institutions did not allow citizens to effectively challenge the legality of the laws and regulations issued by local governments, the weak judicial institutions contributed to the effective functions of the local governments.

Conclusion

This article has explained how the legal and institutional structure of the public health emergency management system has operated between the two stages of "a-securitization" and "hyper-securitization" during the Covid-19 outbreak. It has sought to reveal that China's a-securitization process occurred against its legal inconsistencies and fragmented "*tiao-kuai*" institutions, while the hyper-securitization measures were made possible by the flexibility and responsiveness of its legal system and institutional structure to overcome bureaucratic and hierarchical fragmentation. In this sense, there arises an ironic phenomenon of the Chinese legal and institutional structure of the public health management in China—that is, while the legal vagueness and inconsistency may create belated initial responses to prevent the spread of a public health emergency, they also provide dynamics and flexibility, which allow local governments to effectively address the public health emergency at the later stage.

As this chapter also explains, however, some of the local governments' regulations and actions might have brought about unnecessary fear and panic of citizens, which were not under effective judicial review. It is still uncertain whether, and to what extent, the Chinese legal and institutional structure of the public health emergency management will be reformed, but the Chinese central government has realized the disadvantages of the overuse of the wartime rhetoric. Since April 2020, while sporadic cases were reported in some regions across China, the local infections of Covid-19 were basically under control. However, some regions still reported an entrance into a "wartime mode". For instance, during January 2–4, 2021, a province surrounding Beijing, Hebei Province, reported 19 local infections. It was nearly 6 months after this province reported locally transmitted infections in June 2020. Nationally, on January 4, 2021 the NHC reported 17 local infections with 14 in Hebei. The Hebei government thus entered into the "wartime mode". Apart from Hebei Province, other local governments also widely used an entrance into the "wartime mode". On January 16, 2021, Xinhua News, a Chinese official criticized the local governments' overuse of the wartime mode, by saying that "abusing the expression of 'wartime state' may create unnecessary panic, easily paralyzing the people's psychology and diluting people's awareness of 'war preparation'". It perceives the local governments' overuse of the wartime mode reactions as a "lazy approach" ("lanzheng") (Xinhua News 2020). This suggests that the central government has realized the limitations of the local governments' over-uses of the securitization measures as rhetoric devices, but it also needs to fundamentally improve the institutional and legal structure of the public health emergency management in China in order to avoid the disproportionate effects of increasing the panic of citizens.

Bibliography

Buzan, Barry, Ole Wœver and Jaap de Wilde, *Security: A New Framework for Analysis* (Boulder, CO: Lynne Rienner Publishers, 1998).

Caixin, "Zhongguo Neidi Sanshiyi Shengfen Quanbu Qidong Tufa Gonggong Weisheng Shijian Yiji Xiangying," "中国内地31省份全部启动突发公共卫生事件一级响应," 2020. https://china.caixin.com/2020-01-29/101509411.html.

Coglianese, Cary and Neysun Mahboubi, "Administrative Law in a Time of Crisis: Comparing National Responses to COVID-19," *Administrative Law Review* 73(1) (2021): 1–18.

DeLisle, Jacques and Kui Shen, "China's Response to COVID-19," *Administrative Law Review* 73(1) (2021): 19–52.

Elbe, Stefan, "Pandemics on the Radar Screen: Health Security, Infectious Disease and the Medicalization of Insecurity," *Political Studies* 59(4) (2011): 848–866.

Fidler, David, *SARS, Governance and the Globalization of Disease* (New York: Palgrave, 2004).

Houston, Cameron, "'No Justification': Anger over Mobile Public Surveillance Units at Public Parks," *The Age*, September 6, 2020.

Huang, Yanzhong, *Governing Health in Contemporary China* (Milton Park, Abingdon, Oxon; New York: Routledge, 2013).

Lieberthal, Kenneth and Michel Oksenberg, *Policy Making in China: Leaders, Structures, and Processes* (Princeton: NJ: Princeton University Press, 1988).

Li, Liming et al., "Yiqing Zaoqi, Jibing Yufangkongzhi Tixi Shisheng Yuanyin Hezai?," "疫情早期, 疾病预防控制体系失声原因何在?," Zhishifenzi, 知识分子, http://zhishifenzi.com/depth/depth/8392.html.

Liu, Peng, Xiao Zhong and Suyang Yu, "Striking a Balance between Science and Politics: Understanding the Risk-Based Policy-Making Process during the Outbreak of COVID-19 Epidemic in China," *Journal of Chinese Governance* 5(2) (2020): 198–212.

Lo, Catherine Yuk-Ping, *HIV/AIDS in China and India: Governing Health Security* (New York: Palgrave, 2015).

McInnes, Colin, "The Many Meanings of Health Security," in Simon Rushton and Jeremy Youde (eds.), *Routledge Handbook of Global Health Security* (Milton Park, Abingdon, Oxon; New York, New York: Routledge, 2015): 7–17.

Nelson, Christopher, Nicole Lurie, et al., *Conceptualizing and Defining Public Health Emergency Preparedness* (Arlington, VA: Rand Corporation, 2008).

Norton Rose Fulbright, "Contact Tracing Apps: A New World for Data Privacy," https://www.nortonrosefulbright.com/en-cn/knowledge/publications/d7a9a296/contact-tracing-apps-a-new-world-for-data-privacy#China.

Saich, Tony, "SARS and China's Economy," in Arthur Kleinman and James L. Watson (eds.), *SARS in China: Prelude to Pandemic?* (Stanford, CA: Stanford University Press, 2006): 71–104.

She, Jingwei, "China Gets Top Mark as Citizens Rank Their Governments' Response to the COVID-19 Pandemic: Blackbox Research," 2020, https://news.cgtn.com/news/2020-05-08/Survey-shows-China-s-response-to-COVID-19-gets-top-mark-among-public-Qk5KbpG78k/index.html.

Sina Net, "Hubei Duodi Xuanbu 'Zhanshi Guanzhi', Zhuanjia Cheng Buying Lanyong Gainian," "湖北多地宣布'战时管制', 专家称不应滥用概念", 2020. https://news.sina.cn/gn/2020-02-14/detail-iimxyqvz2903150.d.html.

Sliwinski, Krzysztof, "'A-Securitization' of Immigration Policy—The Case of European Union," *Asia-Pacific Journal of EU Studies* 14(1) (2016): 25–56.

Sohu News, "Zhongyang Lingdaozu Shouci Pilou, Shiyi Wei Buji Ganbu zai Hubei Yixian Xietiao Zhihui," "中央领导组首次披露!11位部级干部在湖北一线协调指挥,", 2020. https://www.sohu.com/a/378422340_120053683.

South China Morning Post, "Street by Street, Home by Home: How China used Social Controls to Tame an Epidemic," 2020. https://www.scmp.com/

news/china/society/article/3080912/wuhans-elderly-reminded-life-under-mao-during-coronavirus.

Stern, Jessica, "Dreaded Risks and the Control of Biological Weapons," *International Security* 27(3) Winter 2002/03.

Stivas, Dionysios and Krzysztof Sliwinsk, "Securitizing Coronavirus: Global Risks, Responses, and Consequences," 2020. https://www.21global.ucsb.edu/global-e/september-2020/securitizing-coronavirus-global-risks-responses-and-consequences.

The Guardian. "Trump Says China Could Have Stopped Covid-19 and Suggest US Will Seek Damages," 2020. https://www.theguardian.com/world/2020/apr/28/trump-says-china-could-have-stopped-covid-19-and-suggests-us-will-seek-damages.

The State Council Information Office of the People's Republic of China, *Fighting Covid-19 China in Action* (Beijing: Foreign Language Press, 2020).

United Nations Development Program (UNDP), Human Development Report 1994, (New York, Oxford: Oxford University Press, 1994).

Wei, Furong et al. "Wuhan Yiqing Chuqi, Wangluo Zhibao Xitong Weihe Shiling," "武汉疫情初期，网络直报系统为何失灵," Phoenix New Media, 2020. https://news.ifeng.com/c/7uqH6A5PWt7.

Xinhua News, "Xi Focus: Chronicle of Xi's Leadership in China's War Against Coronavirus," 2020. http://www.xinhuanet.com/english/2020-09/07/c_139349538.html.

Xinhuawang (新华网) [XINHUANET], "Lanyong 'Zhanshi Zhuangtai' Buliyu Kangyi Daju, 'Langlaile' hui Mabi Qunzhong," (滥用'战时状态'不利于抗疫大局, '狼来了'会麻痹群众), 2021. http://www.xinhuanet.com/politics/2021-01/16/c_1126989719.html.

Yang, Hai, "Wuhan Zaoqi Yiqing Weihe Yidu Zhongduan," "武汉早期疫情上报为何一度中断," Zhongguo Qingnian Bao, 中国青年报, 2020. https://news.sina.cn/gn/2020-03-05/detail-iimxyqvz8101965.d.html.

Yu, Qin and Li Shiyun, 2020. "Zhuangfang Weijianwei Wuhan Dierpi Zhuanjia," "专访卫健委派武汉第二批专家：为何没发现人传," Caijing Zazhi, 财经杂志, 2020. https://news.sina.cn/gn/2020-02-26/detail-iimxxstf4577244.d.html?from=wap.

Index

C. Zhang (ed.), *Human Security in China*,
https://doi.org/10.1007/978-981-16-4675-1

The manufacturer's authorised representative in the EU is Springer Nature Customer Service Centre GmbH, Europaplatz 3, 69115 Heidelberg, Germany. If you have any concerns regarding our products, please contact ProductSafety@springernature.com

Printed and bound by CPI Group (UK) Ltd, Croydon, CR0 4YY
30/09/2026
02225457-0004